GRIEVING THE LIVING

Coping with Grief and Loss While Loving Someone with Dementia

Nadia Wells

This book is for Frank—never forgotten.

Forward

Loving and caring for someone with dementia is one of the most profound and heart-wrenching journeys you can experience. It's a path filled with small, beautiful moments and overwhelming loss—where love deepens even as memories fade.

For me, this journey began with my father. I watched, year after year, as the man I had always known—strong, capable, endlessly resourceful—slowly changed. The hands that once fixed everything now fumbled over the simplest tasks. The gentle, patient man began showing increasing frustration and anger, which was completely out of character. We realized that his change in behavior stemmed from confusion. It was heartbreaking. And it was lonely.

This book was born from that place—of love, of grief, of witnessing. It's for the carers. The spouses, daughters, sons, and friends who show up every day with love in their hearts, even when that love becomes stretched thin by exhaustion, sadness, and uncertainty. It's for those who grieve not just the person their loved one once was, but the future they imagined, the plans they made, the shared memories slowly slipping away.

Some days will feel like a gift. Your loved one might look at you and truly *see* you, and for a moment, you'll feel like nothing has changed. Other days, you may struggle to recognize the person in front of you—or even yourself in this new role. Yet, in between the moments of guilt, fear, and helplessness, sometimes you find a deep peace.

Within my family, my mother bore the greatest weight—physically strong and determined, but grieving too. After more than 60 years of marriage, she was slowly losing her partner in the most painful way imaginable.

This book is for people like her. Like you. I want it to feel like a gentle companion on your shoulder, walking alongside you, supporting you in every step of the journey. Inside, you'll find real-life stories from other carers, insights from grief counselors and nurses, and reflections that I hope bring comfort, understanding, and moments of connection.

You are not alone in this.

Table of Contents

Forward.. iv

Introduction: The Unique Nature of Dementia Related Grief....... 1

Part I - Understanding Dementia and Its Emotional Impact...... 7

Chapter 1: What is Dementia?... 8

Chapter 2: Anticipatory Grief and Ambiguous Loss 18

Chapter 3: The Emotional Rollercoaster 32

Part II - Coping with the Duality of Grief and Love................. 39

Chapter 4: Acknowledging the Loss While Loving the Present 40

Chapter 5: Reconnecting Through the Fog........................ 49

Part III - Moving through Daily Life with Compassion 56

Chapter 6: Building a Supportive Routine 57

Chapter 7: Coping with Challenging Behaviors.................. 65

Chapter 8: Caring for Yourself as You Grieve 71

Part IV - Preparing for the Future While Grieving the Present
.. 83

Chapter 9: Planning for the Next Stage 84

Chapter 10: Coping with the Final Goodbye 95

Part V - Supporting Others... 106

Chapter 11: Helping Family Members Cope..................... 107

Chapter 12: Empowering Friends to Provide Support.......... 121

Part VI - Moving Forward with Love and Resilience............. 129

Chapter 13: Life After Loss 130

Chapter 14: Keeping Their Memory Alive 140

Conclusion: Love and Letting Go................................ 152

A Request 162

Bibliography 163

Appendices **165**

    Appendix A: Essential Resources for Dementia Caregivers 166

    Appendix B: Conversation Starters 167

About the Author **169**

About the Publisher **170**

INTRODUCTION
The Unique Nature of Dementia Related Grief

In 2014, country music legend Glen Campbell embarked on his final tour, after a 50 year career, documented in the poignant film *I'll Be Me*. Despite his Alzheimer's diagnosis, Campbell continued to perform, supported by his family and band.

The tour became a powerful testament to the complexities of dementia-related grief and was particularly significant as it showcased Campbell's resilience and the enduring power of music in the face of cognitive decline.

Audiences witnessed Campbell's musical abilities remain intact even as he struggled with memory and cognition off-stage.

This phenomenon, known as preserved musical memory in Alzheimer's patients, is a well-documented occurrence where those suffering from dementia can often recall and perform music long after other cognitive functions have deteriorated.

His wife, Kim, described the experience as "living grief," mourning the loss of the man she knew while still cherishing the moments of connection through music.

This concept of "living grief" is specifically poignant in cases of dementia, as loved ones must feel their way through the emotional complexity of grieving someone who is still physically present but cognitively changed.

More recently, in 2021, the story of Tony Bennett's final performances with Lady Gaga captured public attention. Despite his advanced Alzheimer's, Bennett performed a full set of songs at Radio City Music Hall.

This remarkable feat further underscored the unique relationship between music and memory in patients with dementia, demonstrating how deeply ingrained musical abilities can be within the brain.

His family and collaborators described the bittersweet nature of these concerts—celebrating Bennett's enduring musical gifts while acknowledging the reality of his condition.

This duality of emotions is a common experience for those caring for dementia sufferers, as they often find themselves oscillating between joy at moments of clarity or connection and sadness at the overall progression of the disease.

By sharing their experiences openly, these celebrities and their families have helped to destigmatize dementia and foster greater understanding of the condition's impact on both patients and caregivers.

These stories illustrate the multifaceted nature of dementia-related grief—a process that combines loss and love, and frustration and joy, often in equal measure.

Moving through this book, we'll look at the various aspects of this emotional battle and talk about strategies for navigating the unique form of loss—but know that you are not alone. It isn't easy ... but as you'll find, you *will* get through this.

Here's a summary of what you can expect to tackle in these pages:

A Different Kind of Loss

Dementia-related grief presents a complex and multifaceted experience that differs significantly from other forms of loss.

When a loved one receives a dementia diagnosis, you may find yourself mourning for the future you had imagined together, for the memories you won't be able to create, and for the gradual loss of the person you've known and loved.

This grief begins long before your loved one's physical death, creating a complex emotional experience to traverse.

One of the most difficult aspects of dementia-related grief stems from its ambiguous nature. Your loved one stays physically present, but their cognitive abilities and personality may change dramatically over time.

Family therapist, Pauline Boss, coined the term "ambiguous loss" in the 1970s to describe this experience of losing someone who is still physically present.

You might find yourself grieving the loss of shared experiences, inside jokes, or the unique connection you once had.

Simultaneously, you're tasked with caring for and supporting your loved one through their changing needs. This duality creates a complex emotional environment where joy, love, grief, and frustration coexist.

Anticipatory Grief: Mourning Future Losses

Anticipatory grief commonly affects those loving someone with dementia.

This type of grief occurs when you begin mourning losses that haven't yet fully materialized. You might grieve for the future decline you know is coming, or for the gradual loss of your loved ones, their abilities and memories.

This anticipatory grief can be particularly challenging because it's ongoing and often unrecognized by others.

You might feel guilty for grieving someone who is still alive, or struggle to explain your emotions to those who don't understand the progressive nature of dementia.

Recognizing that anticipatory grief is a normal and valid response to the ongoing losses associated with dementia can help you cope with the changes as they occur and even help you cherish the moments you have with your loved one in the present.

The Emotional Rollercoaster

Loving someone with dementia often feels like riding an emotional rollercoaster. One day, you might experience a moment of connection that fills you with joy and hope. The next, you might feel overwhelmed by sadness, anger, or frustration as you face a new challenge or loss. These fluctuating emotions are valid and a completely normal part of the experience.

You might experience **sadness** over the gradual loss of your loved one's abilities and memories.

Anger may arise at the unfairness of the disease or the challenges you face.

Guilt might creep in over negative emotions or perceived shortcomings in your caregiving.

Fear about the future and what it holds can be a constant companion.

And yet, **joy** can surprise you in moments of connection or lucidity.

Finally, **love** remains a constant thread, often deepening and taking on new forms as you work your way through this experience together.

Allowing yourself to feel and process these emotions without judgment is important.

Each feeling represents a valid part of your experience and can provide valuable insights both into your needs and those of your loved one.

Shifting Family Dynamics

Dementia affects not just the person diagnosed, but the entire family system.

Your relationships with other family members may change as you manage caregiving responsibilities and differing opinions on care decisions. Siblings who were once close might find themselves at odds over care choices. Adult children might struggle to accept the role reversal as they become caregivers for a parent and spouses might grapple with the loss of their partner and confidant.

These changing dynamics add another layer of complexity to your grief.

Open communication with family members, seeking support when needed, and remembering that everyone grieves and copes differently can help you to brave these challenges.

Finding Meaning and Growth

While the experience of loving someone with dementia undoubtedly challenges you, many also find opportunities for personal growth and deeper connection.

You might explore strengths you didn't know you had, develop a deeper capacity for compassion, or find new ways to express love and care.

This experience might lead you to reassess your priorities and values, potentially leading to positive changes in other areas of your life. Some explore a passion for advocacy or find meaning in supporting others on similar paths.

While it's important not to minimize the difficulties, recognizing and nurturing these opportunities for growth and finding meaning can provide much-needed hope during challenging times.

Your willingness to engage with these difficult emotions and experiences shows the depth of your love and commitment. While each person's experience is unique, the disease is well understood and there are many (including myself) who understand.

By taking care of yourself, seeking support when needed, and finding moments of joy and connection amidst the challenges, you can get through this complex experience with resilience and grace, ensuring every moment counts.

Part I – Understanding Dementia and Its Emotional Impact

CHAPTER 1

What is Dementia?

Dementia affects millions of people worldwide, yet many struggle to fully understand its nature and impact. This chapter explores dementia, its various types, and how it progresses.

You'll learn to recognize the differences between dementia and normal aging, equipping you with knowledge to better support your loved ones affected by this condition.

Understanding Dementia

Dementia describes a decline in cognitive function severe enough to interfere with daily life. It involves loss of memory, language skills, problem-solving abilities, and other cognitive skills that affect a person's ability to perform everyday activities.

Dementia is caused by damage to brain cells, disrupting their ability to talk with each other. This disruption affects thinking, behavior, and feelings.

Contrary to what many believe, dementia isn't a normal part of aging. While more common in older adults, it's not an inevitable consequence of growing older.

Types of Dementia

Several types of dementia exist, each with unique characteristics and causes:

1. Alzheimer's Disease: The most common form, accounting for 60-80% of cases and is caused by an abnormal protein buildup in the brain, leading to brain cell death.

2. Vascular Dementia: The second most common type, caused by reduced blood flow to the brain, often because of small strokes.

3. Lewy Body Dementia: Characterized by abnormal deposits of a protein called alpha-synuclein in the brain.

4. Frontotemporal Dementia: Caused by progressive cell degeneration in the brain's frontal and temporal lobes.

5. Mixed Dementia: Occurs when a person has more than one type of dementia simultaneously.

Understanding these different types helps you comprehend the specific challenges your loved ones might face and the care they might need.

The Nature of Change in Dementia

Dementia affects various regions of the brain, leading to a diverse array of symptoms that alter cognition, behavior, and emotional responses. These changes stem from complex neurological processes beyond your loved one's control.

Understanding this biological basis allows you to approach these changes with greater compassion and patience.

Memory loss often begins with difficulty recalling recent events, while long-term memories remain intact. As the disease advances, even deeply ingrained memories may fade.

You might notice your loved one struggling to recognize familiar places or losing track of time, dates, and seasons.

Cognitive challenges extend beyond memory. Problem-solving, planning, and decision-making abilities may decline, making everyday tasks increasingly difficult.

Your loved one might find it harder to follow conversations, express thoughts clearly, or find the right words.

Personality shifts can be particularly jarring. You may observe changes in mood, increased anxiety or agitation, or behaviors that seem out of character.

These alterations are symptoms of the disease, not choices your loved one is making.

The Progression of Dementia

Dementia typically develops slowly and gradually worsens over time. The rate of progression varies widely from person to person and depends on many factors, including the underlying cause.

Generally, dementia progresses through three stages:

Early Stage

In this stage, a person may function independently, but experience memory lapses.

They might forget familiar words or the location of everyday objects.

Difficulty performing complex tasks or planning may also occur.

Middle Stage

This stage is typically the longest and can last for many years. As the condition progresses, the person may have greater difficulty performing routine tasks and may start forgetting significant details about their life.

Late Stage

In the final stage of dementia, patients lose the ability to respond to their environment, carry on a conversation, and eventually control movement. They may still say words or phrases, but communicating becomes significantly more difficult.

Each person's experience with dementia is slightly varied. Some may experience a rapid decline, while others may live with the condition for many years.

Impact on the Person and Family

Dementia has a profound effect on both the diagnosed and their family.

As the condition progresses, the patient with dementia needs increasing levels of care and support. This can place significant emotional, physical, and financial strain on family members.

For the person with dementia, the impact can include:

- Loss of independence
- Confusion and disorientation
- Changes in personality and behavior
- Difficulty communicating
- Emotional distress, including anxiety and depression
- Difficulty eating and swallowing
- Incontinence
- Loss of mobility

Family members often face challenges such as:

- The emotional toll of watching a loved one change
- The stress of providing care or finding appropriate care
- Adapting to changing needs, both physically and mentally
- Financial burdens associated with care and treatment
- Understanding complex healthcare and legal systems

- Balancing caregiving responsibilities with other life commitments

Understanding these impacts helps you prepare for what lies ahead and seek suitable support when needed.

Recognizing Dementia vs. Normal Aging

As we age, it's normal to experience some changes in cognitive function. However, significant differences exist between normal aging and dementia. Recognizing these differences helps identify potential concerns early so that you can seek suitable medical advice.

Here's a comparison of normal aging versus dementia symptoms:

Normal Aging vs Dementia

- Occasionally forgetting names or appointments vs Forgetting recently learned information or important dates

- Making occasional errors while managing finances vs Difficulty managing finances or solving problems

- Sometimes having trouble finding the right word vs Frequent problems with speech or writing

- Occasionally feeling sad or moody vs Persistent changes in mood or behavior

- Needing occasional help with electronic devices vs Difficulty completing familiar tasks at home or work

- Vision changes related to cataracts vs Difficulty judging distances or determining color

- Slower to learn new things vs Inability to retain new information

Everyone experiences aging differently, and some changes in memory or cognitive skills can be part of the normal aging process. However, if you notice significant changes or if these changes interfere with daily life, speak to a healthcare professional.

Risk Factors and Prevention

While age is the greatest known risk factor for dementia, it's not an inevitable part of aging.

Other risk factors include:

- Family history
- Cardiovascular health
- Education level
- Head injuries
- Excessive alcohol use
- Lack of physical exercise

Some risk factors, like age and genetics, can't be changed. However, research suggests that modifying other risk factors potentially reduces the risk of developing dementia.

To potentially reduce dementia risk, consider implementing these strategies:

1. **Stay Physically Active:** Regular exercise improves blood flow to the brain and reduces the risk of cardiovascular problems linked to dementia.

2. **Maintain a Healthy Diet:** A diet rich in fruits, vegetables, whole grains, and lean proteins may help protect brain health.

3. **Stay Mentally Active:** Engage in activities that challenge your brain, such as learning a new language, doing crosswords and other word-related games, or playing musical instruments.

4. **Stay Socially Connected:** Social engagement may support brain health and reduce the risk of depression, a risk factor for dementia.

5. **Manage Cardiovascular Risk Factors:** Control high blood pressure, high cholesterol, and diabetes.

6. **Get Quality Sleep:** Adequate sleep is necessary for brain health and may help reduce the risk of cognitive decline.

7. **Avoid Excessive Alcohol Consumption and Don't Smoke:** Both have been linked to an increased risk of dementia.

While these steps may help reduce the risk of dementia, they don't guarantee prevention. If you're concerned about cognitive changes in yourself or a loved one, your first step is to always ask a healthcare professional.

Supporting Someone with Dementia

Caring for someone with dementia needs patience, understanding, and a supportive approach.

Here are some strategies to help manage challenging situations:

1. **Establish a Routine:** Create a daily schedule to provide structure and reduce confusion.

2. **Simplify Tasks:** Break complex activities into smaller, manageable steps.

3. **Enhance Communication:** Speak clearly, use simple language, and maintain eye contact.

4. **Create a Safe Environment:** Remove potential hazards and confirm the living space is dementia-friendly.

5. **Encourage Independence:** Allow the person to do as much as they can on their own, offering support when needed.

6. **Use Memory Aids:** Implement visual cues, labels, and reminders to help with daily tasks.

7. **Manage Behavioral Changes:** Understand that challenging behaviors are often a form of communication and respond with patience and empathy.

Understanding dementia is the first step in conquering the challenging path of caring for a loved one with this condition. By recognizing the signs, understanding the progression, and knowing the differences between normal aging and dementia, you can better prepare to provide support and seek help when needed.

While dementia presents significant challenges, it doesn't define the sufferer.

Your loved one is still there, behind the symptoms of the disease. However, it is their mind and the person they once were that is changing.

With knowledge, patience, and compassion, you can continue to connect with them and provide the care and support they need, whilst still creating memories. From personal experience, continue to take photos and videos of your time with your loved one as these become invaluable once they are gone.

CHAPTER SUMMARY

15 Key Points to Understanding and Supporting Those with Dementia

1. **Recognize dementia as a group of cognitive disorders.** Dementia isn't a single disease, but a term covering various conditions affecting brain function.

2. **Understand the most common types of dementia.** Familiarize yourself with Alzheimer's, vascular dementia, Lewy body dementia, and frontotemporal dementia to better support your loved one.

3. **Learn the three stages of dementia progression**. Knowing the early, middle, and late stages helps you anticipate and prepare for changes in your loved one's condition.

4. **Identify the differences between normal aging and dementia.** Learn to distinguish between age-related changes and potential signs of dementia to seek help early if needed.

5. **Recognize the impact of dementia on the person.** Understand how dementia affects independence, communication, and emotional well-being to provide suitable support.

6. **Acknowledge the impact on family caregivers.** Be aware of the emotional, physical, and financial challenges faced by those caring for someone with dementia.

7. **Create a safe and supportive environment.** Remove potential hazards and adapt the living space to accommodate your loved one's changing needs.

8. **Establish consistent routines and simplify tasks.** Provide structure and break down complex activities to help your loved one maintain independence for as long as possible.

9. **Enhance communication with clear language.** Speak slowly, maintain eye contact, and use visual cues to improve understanding and reduce frustration.

10. **Use memory aids and visual reminders.** Implement labels, calendars, and other visual cues to help your loved one manage daily tasks.

11. **Encourage physical activity and social engagement.** Regular exercise and social interaction can help maintain cognitive function and improve overall well-being.

12. **Maintain a healthy diet and manage cardiovascular risk factors.** A balanced diet and control of conditions like high blood pressure can potentially reduce the risk of dementia progression.

13. **Promote mental stimulation through engaging activities.** Encourage puzzles, reading, or learning new skills to help maintain cognitive function.

14. **Manage behavioral changes with patience and empathy.** Understand that challenging behaviors are often a form of communication and respond with compassion.

15. **Prioritize self-care as a caregiver.** Take care of your own physical and emotional health to better support your loved one with dementia.

CHAPTER 2
Anticipatory Grief and Ambiguous Loss

When someone you love receives a dementia diagnosis, you experience emotional turmoil unlike any other. Your loved one stands before you, yet you're acutely aware they're slipping away.

This mix of presence and absence often leaves you feeling confused, sad, and even guilty. Guilt can stem from the desire to do more, yet feeling time-poor, from how your own wellbeing suffers and how emotionally draining caring for a loved one can be, or guilt can also stem from frustration over your loved one's inability to remember things.

Many caring for someone with dementia experience what is called "anticipatory grief" and "ambiguous loss". These terms describe very real and often overwhelming emotions that come with loving someone who is changing because of dementia.

Anticipatory grief involves mourning for losses that haven't happened yet, but that you know are coming. With dementia, you might grieve for future conversations you'll no longer have, memories you won't be able to share, or plans that now seem impossible.

Ambiguous loss describes the confusing state of loving someone who is physically present but psychologically changing or absent. Your loved one is still here, but in many ways, they're not the person you once knew.

These experiences can feel incredibly isolating.

You might think you're the only one going through this, or that no one else could possibly understand.

But these feelings are common, valid, and deserve attention and care.

Anticipatory Grief

Anticipatory grief manifests in many ways when caring for someone with dementia:

Sadness often creeps in when you think about how your loved one won't attend future family events. This sadness can be particularly acute as you imagine milestones like weddings, graduations, or births that your loved may miss or not fully comprehend.

The realization that shared experiences and memories will become increasingly one-sided can be deeply painful. You might feel anxious about the increasing care they'll need as the disease progresses.

This anxiety often stems from uncertainty about the future, concerns about your ability to provide adequate care, and worries about the financial and emotional toll of long-term caregiving.

The gradual loss of your loved one's mental acuity and independence can also trigger fears about your own future and mortality.

Anger at the unfairness of the situation is common, as is guilt for feeling relieved during moments of clarity. The anger may be directed at the disease itself, the healthcare system, or even the person with dementia.

Guilt can arise from various sources, including feeling relief when the person has a good day, frustration with caregiving duties, or regret over past interactions.

All of these feelings are normal.

Acknowledging these emotions can be the first step in learning to cope with them.

Recognizing and accepting these complex feelings without judgment is important for maintaining your own mental health and providing effective care.

It's important to understand that experiencing these emotions doesn't reduce your love or commitment to the person with dementia.

Here's a quick example I'm taking from the personal experience of a friend of mine (Let's just call her Mara):

Mara's Story

Mara sat in the quiet of her mother's living room, the soft scent of lavender lingering in the air. The space felt frozen in time, books still stacked by the reading chair, a forgotten cup of tea growing cold on the windowsill. Upstairs, her mother, June, was resting after a difficult morning. Alzheimer's had slowly rewritten their lives, not all at once, but in pieces, first forgotten appointments, then lost conversations, and now, the fading edges of the woman Mara had always known.

At fifty-three, newly single and with the ability to work remotely, Mara stepped into the role of caregiver without hesitation. June had been her anchor through life's hardest moments, and this felt like a way to honor that bond. But no one had prepared her for the grief that came before the final goodbye, the heartbreak of losing someone who is still right in front of you. Some days brought flickers of clarity: a laugh, a shared memory, a song half-sung from Mara's childhood. Other days, like this one, were filled with questions on repeat, the same conversation circling back again and again. Each time, it chipped away at her strength—and filled her with guilt for feeling so overwhelmed.

That evening, as the sun cast long shadows across the kitchen floor, June looked up from the couch and asked, "Are we having breakfast soon?" Mara had answered that question more times than she could count that day. She paused, her hands still wet from dishes, her heart aching with the weight of love, fatigue, and sorrow. This was the rhythm of her life now, small moments of connection followed by deep waves of loss. In those in-between spaces, Mara grieved not only what was gone but what was still yet to be lost.

She initially felt guilty for grieving, but as she learned more about anticipatory grief, she realized her feelings were a natural response to a difficult situation.

Mara's experience is common among caregivers who often struggle with the concept of grieving someone who is still alive. Understanding anticipatory grief can help caregivers recognize that their feelings are valid and shared by others in similar situations.

Recognizing this helped her be kinder to herself and more present for her mother. By acknowledging and accepting her feelings, Mara was able to reduce her self-criticism and emotional turmoil.

This self-compassion allowed her to focus more energy on quality time with her mother, rather than being consumed by guilt or trying to suppress her emotions.

Ambiguous Loss

Family therapist Pauline Boss coined the term "ambiguous loss" to describe a loss that occurs without closure or clear understanding. With dementia, it's the experience of having someone physically present but psychologically changed or absent.

This concept is particularly relevant in cases of cognitive decline, where a loved one's personality and memories may gradually fade while their physical form remains.

The ambiguity arises from the disconnect between the person's physical presence and their altered mental state, resulting in a complicated emotional state for caregivers and family members.

This type of loss can be particularly challenging because it's ongoing and often gradual. Unlike sudden losses, such as those caused by accidents or acute illnesses, ambiguous loss in dementia unfolds over an extended period, sometimes spanning years or even decades.

This prolonged nature of the loss can lead to chronic stress and emotional fatigue for those involved in the care and support of the affected individual.

There's no clear *before* and *after*, no definitive endpoint. In contrast to other forms of loss where there's a distinct moment of change or departure, ambiguous loss in dementia blurs these lines. The person with dementia may have good days and bad days, moments of lucidity interspersed with periods of confusion, making it difficult for loved ones to pinpoint when the "loss" truly began or when it might end.

The loss continues to advance over time, and as the dementia progresses, new aspects of the person's identity and capabilities may be affected, leading to a series of ongoing losses. This continuous evolution of the condition means that caregivers and family members must constantly adapt to new challenges and grieve new losses, even as they're still processing previous changes.

Traditional grieving rituals don't apply to this situation. You can't have a funeral for someone who's still alive. This lack of socially recognized rituals for ambiguous loss can leave those experiencing it feeling isolated and unsure of how to process their emotions.

The absence of clear cultural or social guidelines for experiencing this type of loss can exacerbate feelings of confusion and helplessness, and others might not recognize or confirm your loss. The invisible nature of cognitive decline, especially in its early stages, can lead to a lack of understanding from those not directly involved in the care of the person with dementia.

This lack of recognition can intensify feelings of isolation and invalidate the very real grief experienced by caregivers and family members. They might say things like, "At least they're still with you," not understanding the complexity of your emotions or the disease.

Such well-intentioned but misguided comments can minimize the profound sense of loss experienced by those dealing with a loved one's cognitive decline. These remarks fail to acknowledge the emotional toll of witnessing the gradual disappearance of a person's essence while their physical form stays.

Validation and Support

One of the challenges of anticipatory grief and ambiguous loss is that others may not understand or recognize your grief.

Seeking out others who can understand your experience is helpful. Support groups for caregivers of patients with dementia can be invaluable.

Online forums or communities often provide a safe space to share your feelings.

Friends or family members who are going through similar experiences can offer understanding and empathy. Mental health professionals specializing in grief and loss can provide professional guidance and support.

Your feelings are valid, and you deserve support and understanding as you maneuver your way through this difficult time.

Ambiguous loss can leave you feeling stuck, unable to move forward because the loss isn't final or clear-cut. It's a state of limbo that can be emotionally exhausting and confusing.

This sense of being trapped between hope and grief can lead to decision-making paralysis, relationship strain, and difficulty in planning for the future.

The Double Loss

One of the cruelest aspects of dementia is the feeling that you lose your loved one twice: once to the disease, and again when they pass away. This double loss can compound your grief and make the emotional feedback even more complex.

The first loss occurs gradually as the disease progresses, eroding the person's memory, cognitive abilities, and often, their personality.

This slow decline can be particularly painful as you witness the person you love slowly slip away, even though they are still physically present. You may find yourself mourning the loss of inside jokes, shared experiences, or the ability to reminisce about past events. The gradual disappearance of personality traits that made your loved one unique are particularly distressing, as you watch them become a different version of themselves. You might mourn the loss of future plans and dreams.

Dementia often forces a reevaluation of long-held expectations for the future.

Plans for retirement, travel, or simply growing old together may need to be abandoned or significantly altered. This loss of anticipated shared experiences can be deeply painful and may need a process of letting go and adjusting to a new reality.

Some even feel guilt over feeling relief when the physical loss finally occurs. This complex emotion is often unexpected and can be difficult to reconcile. The relief may stem from seeing an end to the loved one's suffering or from the cessation of the demanding caregiving responsibilities.

It's important to recognize that feeling relief doesn't diminish the love you had for the person or negate the grief you're experiencing. It's a natural response to a long and challenging ordeal.

These feelings are incredibly painful, but it's also important to remember they're also a testament to the depth of your love and connection.

You're grieving because you deeply care.

The intensity of your emotional response reflects the strength of your bond with the person who has dementia. It's a reflection of the impact they have on your life and the significance of your relationship.

Open Dialogues and Shared Experiences

One of the most challenging aspects of anticipatory grief is the feeling of isolation it can create. Many caregivers feel unable to express their complex emotions, fearing judgment or lack of understanding from others.

The Anticipatory Grief Dialogue builds on psychiatrist Erich Lindemann's work by acknowledging the communicative and interactive nature of processing grief before a loss and is a structured approach to opening up conversations about your experiences and feelings.

It starts by confiding in a trusted friend, family member, or professional counselor who can serve as your dialogue partner. Explain that you'd like to have regular conversations about your caregiving process and the emotions you're experiencing.

Set aside dedicated time for these dialogues, free from distractions.

During your Anticipatory Grief Dialogue sessions, use prompts to guide your conversation. Some examples might include:

- "Today, I'm struggling with ..."
- "A memory I'm holding onto is ..."
- "I'm afraid of ..."
- "I'm grateful for..."
- "I wish others understood that ..."
- "I feel angry at them because ..."

Be honest and vulnerable in your responses. Allow yourself to express emotions fully, without judgment.

Your dialogue partner's role is primarily to listen and confirm your feelings, not to offer solutions or fix things. These dialogues serve many purposes. They provide a safe outlet for expressing difficult emotions, reduce feelings of isolation, and help you gain clarity about your experiences.

Over time, you may find patterns in your thoughts and feelings, leading to deeper self-awareness and more effective coping strategies.

Redefining Your Relationship

As your loved one's dementia progresses, your relationship with them will inevitably change.

This can be one of the most painful aspects of the process, but it can also offer opportunities for new forms of connection.

Finding new ways to talk becomes essential.

This might involve using touch, music, or shared activities, as opposed to relying on verbal communication. Focusing on the emotional connection as opposed to cognitive abilities can help bridge the gap.

Creating new shared experiences that are manageable for your loved one's current capabilities can bring joy to both of you. Celebrating small moments of connection and clarity when they occur becomes incredibly important.

> Another friend of mine, Jen, whose husband has Alzheimer's, found that music helped them connect even as his verbal skills declined.
> "We used to love dancing together," she said. "Now, even though he can't follow a conversation, his face lights up when I put on our favorite songs. We still have those moments of connection through music."

While your relationship may be different, it can still be meaningful and filled with love.

Anticipatory grief often involves worrying about future losses and challenges. While some preparation is necessary, it's important to balance this with living in the present. Making necessary legal and financial preparations can help reduce some anxiety about the future. If possible, have conversations about future care while your loved one can still join in decision-making. This can give you peace of mind and confirm their wishes are respected.

The Role of Memory

Memory plays a complex role in the grief process for those loving someone with dementia. Memories of the person before their illness can bring comfort and joy. However, these same memories can heighten your sense of loss as you compare them to the present reality.

> Gail wrote to me about her mother, who she created a photo album with. Each photo had captions to detail the significance behind each.
>
> "Mom might not always remember who's in the photos," Gail explained, "but she enjoys looking at them, and it gives us something to talk about. Sometimes it even triggers a memory for her."

Special Considerations

Everyone's experience with dementia and grief is unique. Some situations may need extra care and understanding:

If your loved one has early-onset dementia, where symptoms of dementia begin before the age of 65, you might deal with extra challenges like work responsibilities or caring for children. Also, the financial impact can be significant if the person diagnosed is still of working age. An early onset dementia diagnosis can feel like the ground has been pulled out from beneath a person, dreams, careers, and family plans suddenly clouded by fear, confusion, and loss. For loved ones, it's equally heartbreaking to watch someone so full of life slowly slip away, grieving not only the changes in memory and behavior but the future they imagined together. It disrupts roles within the family, brings emotional exhaustion, and forces difficult decisions long before anyone is ready, leaving everyone mourning the loss of who that person once was—while they are still physically present.

When there were complications in your relationship prior to your partner receiving their diagnosis, you might have conflicting emotions about your role as a caregiver. Old resentments or unresolved issues can resurface, adding another layer of complexity to your grief. Becoming a carer out of necessity rather than choice is an emotional and complex journey—one often marked by guilt, resentment, love, and exhaustion all at once. There's a deep internal conflict between wanting to do the right thing and feeling unprepared or overwhelmed by the daily demands. The caregiver may silently grieve the life they once had, the relationship that has changed, and the freedom they've lost, all while carrying the invisible weight of responsibility. It's a role taken on not with readiness, but with reluctant courage, driven by love, duty, or lack of alternatives.

In these cases, seeking specialized support or counseling can be particularly helpful. A professional who understands the unique challenges of your situation can provide targeted strategies and support.

Impact on Family Dynamics

As discussed earlier, dementia doesn't just affect the person diagnosed—it can change entire family systems.

Roles within the family often shift as caregiving responsibilities are distributed.

Old conflicts might resurface, or new ones emerge as family members cope differently with the situation. Some family members may distance themselves, while others become more involved. These changes can add another layer of stress and grief to an already difficult situation. In some cases when one family member takes on the bulk of caring duties, it can unintentionally create deep rifts and power struggles within the family. Resentment may build, both from the caregiver who feels unsupported and from others who feel shut out or judged for not doing more.

Decisions about care can become battlegrounds, cause communication break down and intensify long-held family dynamics under stress. What begins as an act of love can quickly lead to isolation, misunderstanding, and emotional distance if roles and expectations aren't openly discussed and shared.

Open communication becomes imperative during this time. Regular family meetings to discuss care plans, share feelings, and address any issues can help prevent misunderstandings and resentment.

If conflicts become unmanageable, family counseling can provide a neutral space to work through difficulties and find solutions.

Self-Care and Resilience

Caring for someone with dementia while dealing with anticipatory grief and ambiguous loss can be emotionally and physically exhausting.

Self-care isn't a luxury, it's a necessity.

You can't pour from an empty cup.

Make time for activities that replenish you, whether that's reading a book, taking a walk, or spending time with friends.

Don't feel guilty about taking breaks or asking for help.

Building resilience is important throughout this challenging chapter of your life. Resilience doesn't mean you never feel sad or overwhelmed. Instead, this involves developing the ability to keep going as you navigate these difficult situations.

We'll explore specific strategies of self-care further in the book.

Finding Meaning

Many find that caring for a loved one with dementia, despite its challenges, can be a profound and meaningful experience. It can deepen your capacity for compassion, patience, and love.

Some caregivers find purpose in advocating for better dementia care or supporting other families going through similar experiences. Others learn new strengths they didn't know they had.

Anticipatory grief and ambiguous loss are complex emotional experiences that many face loving someone with dementia. By understanding these concepts, validating your feelings, and developing coping strategies, you can survive this challenging time with greater resilience and compassion—both for your loved one and yourself.

There's no "right" way to grieve.

Your experience is unique, and your emotions are valid.

As you move forward, hold on to the moments of profound connection, love, and even joy that can occur despite the challenges. These moments are the light that can guide you through the darkest times.

CHAPTER 3

The Emotional Rollercoaster

Caring for a loved one with dementia resembles riding an emotional rollercoaster. The ups and downs, twists and turns, and unexpected loops can leave you feeling exhilarated during a moment of connection and completely drained the next.

This chapter explores the complex array of emotions that caregivers often experience, helping you understand that your feelings are normal and shared by many others on similar paths.

Shifting Identities, Roles, and Relationships

Dementia profoundly impacts the entire family system and the relationships within it. As a caregiver, you may grapple with shifts in identity, roles, and the very nature of your relationship with your loved one.

Identity Changes

As dementia progresses, both you and your loved one may experience a shift in identity.

Your loved one might struggle with their sense of self as their memories and abilities change.

You might find your own identity evolving as you take on the role of caregiver.

This transition can be particularly challenging if you're caring for a parent, as the traditional parent-child dynamic is often reversed.

Role Redistribution

The progression of dementia often necessitates a redistribution of roles within the family. You might find yourself taking on responsibilities that your loved one once managed, such as handling finances, making medical decisions, or maintaining the household.

This role reversal can be emotionally taxing and may need a period of adjustment. Especially in the early days of dementia, this could be for both those with dementia who aren't comfortable and resent the role reversal, and those that are now taking on a new role.

Relationship Evolution

Perhaps one of the most profound impacts of dementia is the way it changes relationships. As your loved one's cognitive abilities decline, you may find it increasingly difficult to connect in the ways you once did.

Communication might become challenging, shared activities may no longer be possible, and the emotional intimacy you once shared might feel different.

> "The reality is that you will grieve forever. You will not 'get over' the loss of a loved one—you will learn to live with it. You will heal and you will rebuild yourself around the loss you have suffered. You will be whole again, but you will never be the same. Nor should you be the same, nor would you want to." - Elisabeth Kübler-Ross

Getting through the Grief Cycle

Grief is often associated with death, but for caregivers of patients with dementia, grief can begin long before the physical loss of their loved one.

The grief cycle, as described by Elisabeth Kübler-Ross, a Swiss-American psychiatrist who was a pioneer in near-death studies, includes stages such as denial, anger, bargaining, depression, and acceptance. However, grief is not a linear process, especially in the context of dementia caregiving, and you may find yourself cycling through these stages repeatedly as your loved one deteriorates.

Denial

Initially, you might find yourself in denial about the diagnosis or the severity of your loved one's condition. This can manifest as minimizing symptoms or holding onto unrealistic hopes for improvement. You might catch yourself thinking, "It's just normal aging," or "They'll get better with the right medication."

It's not a bad thing to hope, but when it becomes a crutch, it can result in a dangerous and distorted high of positivity, only for it to come crashing down as the disease progresses.

Anger

As the reality of the situation sets in, you might experience anger. This could be directed at the disease, the healthcare system, or even your loved one. You might feel frustrated with the unfairness of the situation or angry at the lack of effective treatments or care options available.

It's important to acknowledge these feelings and find healthy ways to express them. There are a number of creative, social and spiritual outlets you can try, coupled with exercise, to take care of yourself and avoid hurting anyone in the process of venting these frustrations.

Bargaining

In this stage, you might find yourself making deals with a higher power or searching for ways to slow or reverse the progression of the disease. This can lead to exhaustive research into treatments or lifestyle changes.

You might think, "If I just find the right supplement or therapy, things will improve."

Depression

As the losses accumulate, feelings of sadness and hopelessness may set in. This is a natural response to the ongoing grief you're experiencing. You might feel overwhelmed by the challenges of caregiving or mourn the future you had envisioned with your loved one.

Acceptance

Acceptance doesn't mean you're happy about the situation, but rather that you've come to terms with the reality of it. In dementia caregiving, acceptance might involve finding ways to cherish the present moment and adapting to new ways of connecting with your loved one. You might focus on creating meaningful experiences within the limitations of the disease.

These stages can be experienced in any order, and you may revisit certain stages many times throughout your caregiving chapter. This is entirely normal and part of the process of adjusting to the ongoing changes brought about by dementia.

Strategies for Emotional Self-Care

The emotional challenges of dementia caregiving demand intentional self-care. Here are some strategies to help you manage your emotions and maintain your well-being:

Acknowledge Your Feelings

Give yourself permission to feel whatever emotions arise.

Suppressing or denying your feelings can lead to increased stress and burnout.

Keep a journal to track your emotions and identify patterns or triggers.

Practice Mindfulness

Mindfulness techniques can help you stay grounded in the present moment, reducing anxiety about the future and regret about the past. Try simple exercises, like focusing on your breathing for a few minutes each day or using a mindfulness app for guided meditations.

Maintain Your Own Identity

While caregiving may be a significant part of your life, it's just as necessary to maintain other aspects of your identity. Continue pursuing hobbies, maintaining friendships, and engaging in activities that bring you joy.

Set aside time each week for activities that are just for you.

Practice Self-Compassion

Be kind to yourself.

Recognize that you're doing the best you can in a challenging situation.

Treat yourself with the same compassion you would offer a friend in your position.

When you make mistakes or feel overwhelmed, remind yourself that you're human and doing a difficult job.

Engage in Physical Activity

Regular exercise can help reduce stress, improve mood, and boost overall well-being.

Even short walks or gentle stretching can make a difference.

Try to incorporate movement into your daily routine, even if it's just a 10-minute walk around the block.

The Impact of Emotional Intelligence on Caregiving

Understanding and managing your emotions can significantly impact the quality of care you provide and your overall well-being as a caregiver. Here's how:

Enhanced Communication

When you're in tune with your own emotions, you're better equipped to talk effectively with your loved one, healthcare providers, and other family members. This can lead to improved care coordination and a more supportive caregiving environment.

Improved Decision-Making

Emotional awareness helps you make more balanced decisions. By recognizing when you're feeling overwhelmed or frustrated, you can take a step back and approach decisions with a clearer mind.

Increased Empathy

Managing your own emotions allows you to be more present and empathetic with your loved one. This can lead to more meaningful interactions and a deeper connection, even as the disease progresses.

Reduced Burnout Risk

By acknowledging and addressing your emotional needs, you're less likely to experience caregiver burnout. This means you can provide care for longer periods without compromising your own health and well-being.

Better Stress Management

Understanding your emotional triggers helps you develop more effective stress management strategies, which can lead to improved physical and mental health outcomes for you as a caregiver.

How to Move Forward

The emotional mission of caring for a loved one with dementia is complex and challenging. It's a path marked by profound love, deep grief, and everything in between.

By understanding and acknowledging the range of emotions you may experience, you can better weather this ordeal. Practicing self-care, seeking support, and cultivating emotional flexibility can build resilience and enable you to find moments of joy and connection amidst the challenges.

Your emotional well-being is just as important as the physical care you provide. By taking care of yourself emotionally, you're better equipped to provide the best possible care for your loved one.

Part II – Coping with the Duality of Grief and Love

CHAPTER 4

Acknowledging the Loss While Loving the Present

Loving someone with dementia needs constant adaptation and emotional resilience. As the disease progresses, you'll go through a ton of gradual changes, each bringing unique challenges and opportunities for connection.

This chapter explores how to balance acknowledging the losses inherent in dementia while embracing the present moment and the person your loved becomes.

Embracing Your Loved One's Current Self

As you work through your grief, shift your focus towards embracing your loved one as they are now. This doesn't mean forgetting who they were but rather finding new ways to connect and appreciate their current self.

Start by celebrating and encouraging the things your loved one can still do. Adapt activities to match their current capabilities or find new pursuits that bring them joy.

For example, if your loved one enjoyed gardening but can no longer manage the physical tasks, involve them in choosing plants or arranging flowers indoors.

Learn to connect through non-verbal cues, touch, or shared activities that don't rely heavily on language. Pay attention to body language and facial expressions as choice forms of communication. A gentle touch or a warm smile can convey love and support when words fail.

Find joy in simple moments. Appreciate small gestures, fleeting smiles, or moments of clarity as precious gifts. These brief connections can be deeply meaningful for both of you.

Cherish a shared laugh over a favorite TV show or the contentment of sitting together in a sunny garden. Practice patience and compassion, remembering that challenging behaviors are often expressions of unmet needs or frustrations. Approach these moments with empathy and try to understand the underlying cause rather than reacting to the behavior itself.

For instance, if your loved one becomes agitated in the evening, they might be experiencing sundowning syndrome, a common symptom of dementia that causes increased confusion and anxiety as daylight fades.

Sundowning syndrome is a common and sometimes distressing symptom in people with dementia, where confusion, agitation, anxiety, or aggression worsen in the late afternoon and evening. For carers, it can be especially challenging time as it often disrupts daily routines and rest, just when you both are already tired. The unpredictability and intensity of sundowning can be emotionally and physically exhausting.

Balancing Past and Present

While accepting your loved one's current reality is important, honoring and preserving memories of the past plays a vital role in maintaining identity and connection.

Like my friend Gail did in an earlier chapter, try preserving old memories or fill boxes with photos, mementos, and stories in a format that's easy for your loved one to engage with. This can serve as a tangible link to their past and a tool for reminiscence.

Regularly share stories about past experiences, even if your loved one doesn't always remember them. The emotional connection can still be meaningful, and you may be surprised by moments of recognition or joy.

Use music and sensory cues to evoke positive memories and emotions. Play favorite songs from their youth or use familiar scents like a beloved perfume or freshly baked cookies to trigger pleasant associations. Or engage in sensory activities that stimulate the senses, such as gardening, cooking, or art projects.

Focus on the process rather than the outcome, allowing for creativity and self-expression.

Spend time in nature by taking walks in the park, sitting in a garden, or simply watching birds at a feeder. Nature can have a calming effect and provide opportunities for shared enjoyment without the pressure of conversation.

Choose activities that match your loved one's current abilities to foster accomplishment and enjoyment.

Creating Meaningful Rituals

Establishing meaningful rituals provides structure, comfort, and simply a source of enjoyment for both you and your loved one with dementia. These rituals create a framework for ongoing love and care that adapts to your changing relationship.

Incorporate small, consistent rituals into your daily routine to provide stability and connection. Start each day with a warm, loving greeting, perhaps accompanied by a gentle touch or hug. This sets a positive tone for the day and reinforces your bond.

Make mealtimes special by setting the table nicely, playing soft music, or sharing a moment of gratitude. This can help create a calm, enjoyable atmosphere, even if eating habits have changed.

Develop a calming bedtime routine, such as reading a short story, listening to soothing music, or simply sitting together quietly. This can help signal the end of the day and promote better sleep.

Larger weekly or monthly rituals provide something to look forward to and create opportunities for more extensive engagement. Take regular outings to familiar places or scenic areas, even if it's just a short drive around the neighborhood. This change of scenery can be stimulating and enjoyable.

Host regular family meals or gatherings, adapting them to your loved one's comfort level and abilities, to maintain important social connections while fostering feelings of belonging.

Choose familiar films or musicals that your loved one enjoys for movie nights, creating a cozy atmosphere for shared entertainment and to possibly evoke positive memories and emotions.

It's important to continue to mark the passage of time and celebrate holidays. Maintain important holiday traditions, adapting them as needed to accommodate your loved one's current abilities, focusing on the aspects that bring the most joy and meaning.

Involve your loved one in simple decorating tasks for each season or holiday, using familiar items that evoke positive memories. A simple cake, a favorite meal, or a small gathering can be deeply meaningful.

This helps orient them to the time of year and creates a festive atmosphere.

However, some days, you or your loved one simply might not be up for it—and that's okay. There will be other moments. Outings and celebrations, while meaningful, can also carry a quiet undercurrent of stress.

As someone who's walked this path, I know the worry that comes with wondering if they'll have an accident, become disoriented, or react in a way that's hard to manage, like refusing to walk, calling out loudly or saying things that are inappropriate.

That doesn't mean you should give up on joy—it just means you can shape it to fit your current reality.

Let go of expectations. Create rituals that work for *you* and for *them*, in ways that feel gentle, flexible, and safe. Even the smallest traditions can hold deep meaning.

Adapting Your Approach as the Disease Progresses

As dementia advances, your approach to care and connection may need to evolve.

Simplify communication by using short, clear sentences and giving one instruction at a time and try not to overwhelm their attention span or processing.

Pay attention to your tone of voice, facial expressions, and body language, as these can convey meaning even when words fail. Also, focus on sensory experiences as cognitive abilities decline. Soft textures, pleasant scents, and soothing sounds can provide comfort and engagement.

It's also important to prioritize comfort and safety by creating an environment that minimizes stress and promotes well-being.

While structure is important, be prepared to adapt when things don't go as planned. Flexibility can help reduce frustration for both of you. As caregiving demands increase, don't forget to prioritize your own well-being. Regular breaks, support from others, and attention to your physical and emotional health are essential.

Practical Exercises for Connection

To reinforce these concepts and strengthen your connection, try incorporating these exercises into your daily routine:

1. **Gratitude Practice**: Each day, write down one thing you appreciate about your loved one in their current state. This helps shift focus to the positive aspects of your relationship.

2. **Sensory Exploration**: Choose an object with interesting textures, scents, or sounds. Explore it together, describing what you observe. This promotes mindfulness and sensory engagement.

3. **Adaptation Workshop**: Select a favorite activity your loved one can no longer do in its original form. Brainstorm ways to adapt it to their current abilities, focusing on the essence of what made it enjoyable.

4. **Memory Sharing**: Set aside time each week to look through old photos or mementos together. Note which items spark recognition or positive emotions and use these as starting points for connection.

5. **Ritual Creation**: Design a new daily or weekly ritual that suits your loved one's current interests and abilities. Implement it for a month, adjusting as needed, and observe its impact on your relationship.

To Love Deeply, Adapt Continuously

Loving someone with dementia needs a delicate balance of honoring the past, embracing the present, and adapting to constant change. By acknowledging your grief, shifting your focus to your loved one, and creating meaningful rituals and connections, you can continue to nurture your relationship and find moments of joy amidst the challenges.

Remember that this ordeal is not one you need to face alone.

Seek support when needed, be gentle with yourself, and celebrate the small victories along the way.

Your love and care make a profound difference in your loved one's life, even if it may not always feel that way.

By continuing to express your love and adapting your approach, you create a legacy of compassion that transcends the boundaries of dementia.

Your unwavering presence and adaptability provide comfort, dignity, and connection in a world that may often feel confusing to your loved one. In this pathway of love and loss, your ability to grow, adapt, and find new ways to connect becomes a powerful testament to the enduring strength of the human heart.

CHAPTER SUMMARY

10 Keys to Acknowledging Loss While Loving the Present

1. **Understand the biological basis of dementia-related changes.** Recognize that alterations in behavior and abilities stem from the disease, not choices. This understanding fosters greater compassion and patience.

2. **Allow yourself to experience anticipatory grief.** Acknowledge the full range of emotions that come with losing aspects of your loved one while they're still present. This process is normal and necessary for acceptance.

3. **Shift focus to your loved one's remaining abilities.** Celebrate and encourage what they can still do as opposed to dwelling on losses. Adapt activities to match their current capabilities.

4. **Learn new ways of non-verbal communication.** Pay attention to body language, facial expressions, and touch as choice forms of connection. These can convey meaning when words fail.

5. **Create a supportive environment tailored to changing needs.** Modify their living space to promote comfort, safety, and independence. Simple changes can significantly reduce confusion and anxiety.

6. **Balance honoring the past with creating new connections.** Use albums and familiar items to maintain identity, while also engaging in new, sensory-rich activities together.

7. **Establish meaningful daily and weekly rituals.** Incorporate consistent routines that provide structure and comfort. These rituals create a framework for ongoing care and connection.

8. **Use music and sensory cues to evoke positive emotions.** Play favorite songs or introduce familiar scents to trigger pleasant associations. These sensory experiences can be powerful tools for engagement.

9. **Practice mindfulness and presence in your interactions.** Focus on the current moment as opposed to past abilities or future worries. This approach enhances the quality of your time together.

10. **Adapt your caregiving approach as the disease progresses.** Remain flexible in your communication and expectations. Prioritize comfort and sensory experiences as cognitive abilities decline.

CHAPTER 5
Reconnecting Through the Fog

Dementia changes a lot about your communication and dynamic with your loved one, but it doesn't erase the core of who they are.

Their personality, preferences, and capacity for joy often continue long after other faculties have faded. By focusing on these enduring qualities, you can forge new pathways of connection and find moments of genuine joy amidst the challenges.

Adapting Your Communication Style

As cognitive abilities decline, traditional methods of interaction may no longer suffice.

However, by adjusting your approach, you can create new avenues for meaningful connection.

Start by **simplifying your language**.

Use short, clear sentences and avoid complex vocabulary.

Speak slowly and clearly, giving your loved one time to process information.

Visual cues like gestures, facial expressions, and objects can help convey meaning when words fall short.

Choose quiet environments for important conversations to minimize distractions and always allow extra time for responses.

Avoid rushing or finishing sentences for them.

When asking questions, **opt for yes/no** options rather than open-ended queries, as these are often easier to answer.

Most importantly, **confirm their feelings**.

Acknowledge their emotions, even if the context seems unclear.

Your understanding and acceptance can provide comfort, even when words fail.

Focusing on Strengths and Personality

I think I've hinted at this in prior chapters, but now's a great time to really play into it.

As dementia progresses, it's natural to grieve the loss of certain abilities or traits. However, by consciously shifting your focus to your loved one, your enduring strengths and core personality, you can maintain a more positive and meaningful connection.

Take time to reflect on the basic qualities that make your loved one unique.

These might include their sense of humor, kindness, creativity, love of nature, spiritual beliefs, or resilience.

By recognizing and nurturing these enduring qualities, you honor the essence of who they are, beyond the limitations imposed by dementia.

Once you've identified these strengths and interests, consider how you can adapt activities to allow these qualities to shine. For the music lover, create playlists of favorite songs or engage in simple music-making activities.

For the nature enthusiast, take short nature walks or bring natural elements indoors.

If your loved one was always a nurturer, introduce a robotic pet or involve them in simple caregiving tasks. For the artist, offer simplified art projects or create a gallery of their work.

If they were a social butterfly, organize small, manageable social gatherings or engage in other outdoor meet-and-greet activities.

By tailoring activities to your loved one's strengths and interests, you create opportunities for them to feel capable, engaged, and valued. This approach can improve mood, reduce agitation, and enhance overall quality of life.

Reframing Expectations

As you focus on your loved one's strengths, it's important to adjust your expectations and redefine what constitutes a meaningful interaction or accomplishment.

Success might look like a moment of shared laughter, a brief display of affection, or engagement in a simple activity, even if not completed.

Celebrate these moments. By shifting your focus from what's been lost to what remains, you foster a more positive and nurturing environment for both your loved one and yourself.

Humor and Spontaneity

Laughter and lightheartedness are powerful tools for connection, even when facing the challenges of dementia. Look for humor in everyday situations, as shared laughter can diffuse tension and create a bond. Don't be afraid to be playful—make funny faces, tell jokes, or engage in gentle teasing if it's well-received.

Develop simple, recurring jokes or phrases that you can share, or bring along props like funny hats or oversized sunglasses to spark laughter and creativity. These can become comforting rituals.

Be open to unexpected moments of joy and seize these opportunities when they arise, and don't take yourself too seriously.

Your loved one may find comfort in seeing you relaxed and able to laugh at your own mistakes.

As Charlie Chaplin said, "A day without laughter is a day wasted."

Preserving Dignity and Autonomy

As cognitive abilities decline, it becomes increasingly important to preserve your loved one's sense of dignity and autonomy. Offer choices whenever possible, even if limited. For example, ask, "Would you like to wear the blue shirt or the green one?" rather than simply dressing them.

Involve them in daily tasks to the extent of their abilities. This might mean asking them to help fold laundry or set the table, even if the results aren't perfect. The sense of purpose and contribution is more important than the outcome.

Always speak to them directly, not about them to others in their presence, and respect their personal space and privacy, especially during personal care tasks.

Acknowledge their feelings and opinions, even if you disagree or if their perspective seems confused.

Claire's Story:

Claire used to tease Jack that he had the patience of a saint—unless he was stuck behind a slow driver. He was steady, kind, and always had a corny pun ready. Forty-seven years of marriage, and he could still make her laugh when she didn't want to. That's part of what made it so hard—watching the man she loved slowly forget the very life they built together.

At first, it was little things. He'd leave the milk in the pantry or forget someone's name at church. They'd both brushed it off with humor—"Just getting old," he'd say. But over time, it became more than that. More confusion. More silence. And more grief, long before any final goodbye.

But she learned to stop chasing the Jack who once was and started embracing the Jack who *still* was. The Jack who still hummed Johnny Cash under his breath when he was content. Who smiled that crooked smile when she wore her red dress—the one he always loved. So, she began finding ways to help those parts of him shine. They'd sit on the porch and listen to country music, and when a favorite came on, he'd tap his fingers on the armrest like he was drumming along. She'd join in with a little two-step, and sometimes he'd laugh and say, "You're still the best dancer I ever saw." Even if he didn't remember her name in that moment, he remembered how she made him feel.

She gave him choices every day—socks with stripes or plain, coffee or tea, even if he didn't always answer. And she still asked for his help. Folding clothes, feeding the cat, watering the plants. Most days, it didn't matter how well the task was done. What mattered was that he felt needed, not forgotten.

Practical Strategies for Reconnection

To help you put these concepts into practice, here's a step-by-step guide for fostering meaningful connections:

1. **Prepare the environment:** Choose a quiet, comfortable space with good lighting. Minimize distractions by turning off the TV and silencing phones. Have any necessary materials ready, such as photos, a music player, or art supplies.

2. **Center yourself:** Take a few deep breaths and set aside your worries. Remind yourself to be patient and present in the moment.

3. **Initiate contact:** Approach from the front, making eye contact. Offer a gentle touch or hug if appropriate. Greet them by name with a warm smile.

4. **Assess their current state:** Observe their mood and energy level. Ask a simple question about how they're feeling. Be prepared to adjust your plans based on their state.

5. **Engage in a shared activity:** Choose something aligned with their interests and abilities. Start with a simple explanation or demonstration. Participate alongside them, offering gentle guidance as needed.

6. **Practice mindful communication:** Speak slowly and clearly, using simple language and short sentences. Allow plenty of time for responses. Use visual cues or gestures to support your words.

7. **Focus on the process, not the outcome:** Emphasize enjoyment over achievement. Offer praise for effort and engagement. Be flexible and willing to change course if needed.

8. **Create moments of connection:** Share a laugh or smile. Offer words of affirmation and love. Engage in gentle physical touch if appropriate.

9. **Wind down thoughtfully:** Give a five-minute warning before ending the activity. Express gratitude for the shared time. Transition gently to the next part of their routine.

10. **Reflect and adjust:** Take a moment to appreciate any positive moments. Consider what worked well and what could be improved. Use these insights to tell future interactions.

Each day and each interaction may be different, so stay flexible, patient, and focused on the core goal of connection and love.

By approaching each interaction with patience, creativity, and an open heart, you honor the essence of your loved one.

Your presence and love make a profound difference, even in the midst of fog and confusion. The bond you share transcends the limitations of dementia, rooted in a lifetime of shared experiences and emotions that stay even when memories fade.

Love is not a memory—it's a feeling that resides in the heart and soul. By nurturing this connection, you enrich your loved one's life and find meaning and moments of joy in your own.

Part III – Moving through Daily Life with Compassion

CHAPTER 6

Building a Supportive Routine

Creating a supportive routine for anyone suffering from dementia provides stability and familiarity in their increasingly confusing world.

A well-structured daily schedule reduces anxiety, improves sleep patterns, and enhances overall quality of life for both the person with dementia and their caregiver.

The Foundation of Effective Care

A consistent daily routine acts as an anchor, offering comfort and predictability.

As cognitive abilities decline, familiar surroundings and activities may suddenly seem strange.

In this context, a regular schedule becomes a powerful tool to reduce confusion and stress.

Routines help those with dementia orient themselves in time and space. This significantly reduces feelings of disorientation and the associated anxiety.

Additionally, routines preserve normalcy and continuity, allowing individuals to maintain a connection to their pre-dementia life and identity.

From a neurological perspective, routines help maintain cognitive function. The repetition of familiar activities reinforces neural pathways, potentially slowing cognitive decline in some areas.

The predictability of routines also reduces cognitive load, allowing them to conserve mental energy for other tasks and interactions.

For caregivers, establishing and maintaining routines provides structure and purpose to their role. It helps manage time more effectively, reduces stress, and creates opportunities for meaningful engagement with their loved ones.

Striking a balance between structure and flexibility is important, as the needs and abilities of patients with dementia change over time.

Benefits of a Structured Day

Reduced Anxiety and Confusion

A consistent daily schedule provides the comfort of predictability, which significantly reduces feelings of anxiety and confusion in sufferers of dementia. When they know what to expect throughout the day, it creates security and comfort.

Improved Sleep Patterns

Regular routines, especially those that include consistent wake and sleep times, help regulate the body's internal clock. This leads to improved sleep quality and duration, which is often a challenge for those with dementia.

Enhanced Independence

Familiar routines allow your loved one to maintain autonomy for longer periods. When tasks are performed regularly in a consistent manner, muscle memory helps them finish these tasks with less assistance.

Smoother Transitions

Moving from one activity to another can be challenging for those with dementia. A set routine makes these transitions smoother and less stressful. Trying things like letting them know that you will move on to the next activity in 5 minutes, will help them prepare for the change.

Cognitive Stimulation

Regular activities incorporated into a routine offer mental engagement and help maintain cognitive function. This can include activities like puzzles, reading, or listening to music.

Emotional Comfort

The familiarity of a routine provides emotional security and comfort. A sense of stability is particularly useful during times of stress or while facing new challenges.

Improved Medication Management

A structured routine helps ensure medications are taken at the right times, which is important for managing symptoms and maintaining overall health.

Creating a Supportive Routine

To build an effective routine, start by observing your loved one's natural rhythms and preferences. Note when they seem most alert, when they prefer to eat or rest, and which activities they enjoy most. Collecting this information will help you build a routine that aligns with their natural tendencies.

Understanding these patterns significantly increases the effectiveness of the routine. If your loved one is most alert in the morning, schedule cognitively demanding activities during this time.

Try to maintain regular times for waking up and going to bed to help regulate the body's internal clock and improve overall sleep quality and consistency.

Schedule regular mealtimes and include healthy snacks between meals. Incorporate familiar foods and family recipes into meal plans to evoke positive memories and provide comfort. Also, proper nutrition is important for overall health and can help manage some dementia symptoms.

Physical activity potentially slows cognitive decline in some patients with dementia, so include regular periods of gentle exercise or movement in the daily routine. This could be a short walk, chair exercises, or gardening, depending on your loved one's abilities.

Aim for at least 30 minutes of moderate activity most days of the week.

Plan activities that engage the mind, such as puzzles, reading, or listening to music to help maintain cognitive function and provide enjoyment. Tailor these activities to your loved one's interests and abilities. For instance, if they enjoyed crossword puzzles in the past, they may find simplified versions engaging and useful.

Include quiet times for rest and relaxation throughout the day. This is especially important if your loved one becomes tired or overwhelmed easily.

Be mindful of signs of fatigue or overstimulation and be prepared to adjust the routine as needed.

Schedule regular times for personal hygiene tasks, such as bathing, grooming, and dressing. These routines help maintain dignity and self-esteem.

Break down these tasks into simple steps and provide gentle guidance as needed to preserve their independence while ensuring proper care.

Simplifying Daily Tasks

As dementia progresses, once simple daily tasks may become challenging for your loved one. Simplify these tasks while still allowing them to maintain as much independence as possible to help preserve their dignity and sense of self-worth.

Dressing Made Easier

Lay out clothes in the order they should be put on and offer limited choices to avoid overwhelming them. Consider using a "clothing station" with everything needed for dressing in one place to make the process more manageable and less confusing. Also, choose clothing with simple fastenings like Velcro or elastic waistbands.

Bathing with Comfort and Safety

Create a consistent bathing routine at the time of day when your loved one is most cooperative.

Prepare everything in advance to make the process smoother and use safety features like non-slip mats and grab bars. Consider using bath products with familiar scents, as this can be comforting and may evoke positive memories.

Mealtime Strategies

Serve meals in a quiet, calm environment and use contrasting colors for place settings to make it easier to distinguish items.

Consider using adaptive utensils and dishes designed for those with dementia or offering finger foods if using utensils becomes difficult, which can help maintain independence during meals.

Grooming with Dignity

Simplify the grooming routine by using electric razors or easy-to-hold hairbrushes.

Break down tasks into simple steps, providing gentle guidance and encouragement.

Toileting with Independence

To establish a regular toileting schedule, place clear signs on the bathroom door and consider using a toilet seat in a contrasting color to make it more visible. Combined with easy-to-remove clothing, these steps can help prevent accidents and maintain independence.

It's important to provide just enough assistance to ensure safety and success, while still allowing your loved one to do as much as they can independently.

Adapting as Needs Change

One of the most challenging aspects of caring for someone with dementia is the constant need for adaptation. As the condition progresses, your loved one's abilities and needs will change, requiring adjustments to their routine and care plan.

Watch for signs that show a need for change. These might include increased confusion or agitation during certain activities they previously enjoyed, difficulty completing once manageable tasks, changes in sleep patterns or appetite, new safety concerns, or shifts in mood or behavior.

To adapt effectively, periodically assess your loved one's abilities and adjust the routine accordingly. This might involve working with healthcare professionals to conduct formal assessments.

Be prepared to change activities or schedules as needed, even on a day-to-day basis. What works one day may not work the next, so maintain an open and adaptable approach.

Continuously look for ways to simplify tasks and routines as abilities decline. This might involve breaking tasks into smaller steps or using adaptive equipment.

Maintain open dialogue with healthcare providers to address changing needs. Regular check-ins help identify new challenges and potential solutions.

Remember to adjust your own routine and self-care practices as caregiving demands change. Caregiver burnout is a real concern, and taking care of yourself is important for providing the best care possible.

Practical Tips for Implementation

When you implement a supportive routine, start small.

Begin by establishing one or two key routines, then gradually build from there to prevent overwhelming both you and your loved one.

Create a visual schedule using pictures or simple words to help your loved one follow the routine. This can be particularly helpful for those who're dealing with declining verbal communication skills.

Try to stick to the routine as much as possible, but allow for flexibility when needed. Consistency helps reinforce the routine, making it more effective over time.

Where possible, include your loved one in planning the routine to give them a feeling of control. This involvement can increase their engagement and cooperation with the routine.

Use cues or signals to help your loved one transition between activities smoothly. This might include verbal prompts, music, or visual cues. Schedule more demanding tasks during times when your loved one is typically alert to ensure tasks are completed successfully and with less frustration.

It may take time for both you and your loved one to adjust to a new routine, so be prepared for setbacks and remember that consistency over time is important.

Acknowledge and celebrate when the routine works well, no matter how small the success. This positive reinforcement can be encouraging for both you and your loved one.

Don't hesitate to ask for help from family members or professional caregivers in maintaining the routine. Having extra support makes the routine more sustainable in the long term.

Key Considerations for Caregivers

Building a supportive routine for someone with dementia needs balance and adaptability.

As always, I stress that flexibility is needed as it allows for adjustments as needs change.

By focusing on creating a routine that supports both the person with dementia and the caregiver, it's possible to get through the challenges of dementia care with greater confidence and effectiveness.

The goal is to create a supportive framework that enhances the quality of life for both you and your loved one.

CHAPTER 7
Coping with Challenging Behaviors

D ementia changes your loved one in ways you never imagined. One day, they're sharing stories over coffee—the next, they're lashing out in confusion. Challenging behaviors become puzzles waiting to be solved. Your loved one desperately tries to talk in a world that's becoming increasingly bewildering.

With the right tools and mindset, you can learn to help them manage these behaviors.

Aggression, **wandering**, **sundowning**—these behaviors often have underlying triggers.

Physical discomfort, environmental factors, or unmet needs frequently spark these reactions.

Your role becomes that of a detective, piecing together clues to understand what's really going on.

Each challenging behavior offers an opportunity to learn and grow together.

As we explore strategies and solutions, remember that what works today might not work tomorrow, and what helps one person might not help another.

Be prepared to adapt, experiment, and sometimes just roll with the punches.

Your toolkit will grow, along with your confidence in handling whatever dementia throws your way.

Creating a Calm Environment

Your loved one's mind often feels like a stormy sea.

Your goal is to create an island of calm amidst that chaos.

Start with their environment.

Clutter, noise, and harsh lighting can disrupt their fragile sense of peace.

Look closely at their living space. Is it soothing or overstimulating?

Begin by decluttering.

Remove unnecessary items that might cause confusion or frustration. That stack of old magazines from years ago?

It's time to let them go.

Organize remaining items in clear, labeled containers. This approach reduces visual chaos and helps your loved one maintain independence by easily finding what they need instead of constant confusion.

Next, address the sensory elements. Soft, warm lighting can work wonders in reducing agitation.

Consider installing dimmer switches or using table lamps instead of harsh overhead lights.

Think about the sounds in their environment too. If the TV constantly blares, replace it with gentle background music or nature sounds.

Even the ticking of a loud clock can be unsettling for someone with dementia.

Temperature matters more than you might think. Patients with dementia often struggle to regulate their body temperature.

Keep the room comfortably warm, but not stuffy, and provide easy access to light blankets or sweaters so they can adjust as needed.

Familiar objects work well towards conserving memory. Surrounding your loved one with cherished photos, favorite blankets, or meaningful trinkets can provide security in an increasingly unfamiliar world.

Specific Challenges

Even with the best preparation, you'll likely encounter some specific challenging behaviors. Let's explore a few common ones:

Wandering

Wandering can be one of the most dangerous behaviors associated with dementia.

Start by ensuring your home is secure. Use door alarms or bells and consider disguising exits with curtains or wallpaper.

Create a safe space for pacing, like a circular path through the house or a secured outdoor area, and provide plenty of physical activity during the day to reduce restlessness.

Consider using GPS tracking devices or identification bracelets in case your loved one manages to leave the house. Inform neighbors and local authorities about you're their condition so they can be on the lookout.

Aggression

When faced with aggressive behavior, your first priority is ensuring your own safety.

Step back and give them space. Speak calmly and avoid confrontation.

Try to identify the trigger—are they in pain? Frustrated? Scared?

Address the underlying need if possible.

Distraction can be a powerful tool. Have a few go-to activities or topics ready to redirect their attention.

This might be looking at a favorite photo album, listening to a beloved song, or engaging in a simple task they enjoy.

The aggression isn't personal. It's a symptom of the disease and often stems from fear or confusion. Maintaining a calm demeanor can help de-escalate the situation.

Sundowning

As evening approaches, create a calm environment to combat sundowning such as reducing noise and activity levels.

Limit caffeine and sugar intake, especially in the afternoon. Increase daytime activities and exposure to natural light to help regulate their sleep-wake cycle. You could also consider using light therapy.

Exposure to bright light during the day and dimmer light in the evening can help regulate sleep patterns. Some caregivers find success with "dawn simulator" alarm clocks that gradually increase light in the morning.

Hallucinations

When your loved one experiences hallucinations, don't argue or try to convince them what they're seeing isn't real. This will only cause frustration and upset them. Instead, acknowledge their feelings and provide reassurance.

You might say, "I know you're scared. You're safe here with me." Then, gently redirect their attention to something tangible in the room.

Ensure the environment is well lit to reduce shadows that may trigger hallucinations. Check for underlying causes like medication side effects or infections, which can sometimes contribute to hallucinations.

As I've mentioned before, what works one day might not work the next. Be prepared to adapt your strategies as needed. Your flexibility and patience are invaluable assets in managing these challenging behaviors.

Additional Strategies for Tricky Situations

Creating a "rummage box" filled with safe, interesting objects for your loved one to explore can be helpful when they're feeling restless. Include items with different textures, colors, and functions. This might include soft fabrics, smooth stones, colorful plastic items, or simple puzzles.

Aromatherapy can promote calm in some, though it's important to be selective with scents. Lavender, for example, has been shown to reduce agitation in some patients with dementia. Use essential oils in a diffuser or apply diluted oils to the skin (always check with a healthcare provider first).

Weighted blankets or lap pads can reduce anxiety for some. The gentle pressure can be soothing, especially during periods of agitation.

Some find comfort in caring for a lifelike doll or stuffed animal. This practice, known as "doll therapy," helps reduce anxiety by giving them something to focus on. However, it's not suitable for everyone, so observe your loved one's reaction carefully.

Simple puzzles or sorting activities can provide mental stimulation and a sense of accomplishment. Choose puzzles with large pieces and simple designs.

Sorting tasks might include organizing colored beads, buttons, or even socks.

Creating an album with photos and short captions can help orient your loved one and spark positive memories. Include pictures of family members, past homes, and favorite activities.

Review the book together regularly and be sure to give them time to process each page.

When to Seek Professional Help

While many challenging behaviors can be managed at home, there are times when professional help is necessary—both for your peace of mind and your loved ones' sake.

Seek medical advice if:

- Behaviors pose a safety risk to the person with dementia or others
- You're unable to manage the behaviors despite trying various strategies
- There's a sudden change in behavior, which could show an underlying health issue
- You're feeling overwhelmed or burned out despite self-care routines

Your loved one's primary care physician can be a good starting point. They may refer you to specialists like geriatric psychiatrists or neurologists who have expertise in managing dementia-related behaviors.

Consider reaching out to organizations like the Alzheimer's Association (or whichever neurological and mental health departments are available in your area). They offer education, support, and resources for those with dementia and their caregivers.

With the right tools and support, you can continue to provide the care and comfort your loved one needs while also taking care of your own well-being.

CHAPTER 8
Caring for Yourself as You Grieve

W e've touched on this early on, as well as the importance (and benefits) of emotional self-care. But in the course of writing this book, I've decided that I'd like to dedicate an entire chapter to an in-depth look at proper self-care strategies.

Acknowledging and addressing your own grief is necessary for maintaining your well-being and providing the best possible care for your loved one. It's a delicate balance—honoring your emotions while meeting the demands of caregiving.

Many caregivers feel guilty about experiencing grief while their loved one is still alive, which is natural and valid.

Recognizing and addressing these feelings can help you provide more compassionate care and maintain your own emotional health in the long run.

Developing Emotional Awareness

To manage caregiver grief effectively, you need to develop strategies for recognizing and coping with your emotions. One powerful approach is to practice self-reflection and emotional awareness.

Start by keeping a journal to track your feelings.

Set aside 10-15 minutes each day to write about your experiences, thoughts, and emotions. Doing this can help you identify patterns in your grief and recognize triggers that intensify your feelings.

Engage in mindfulness exercises to stay present and aware of your emotions without judgment. Simple techniques like deep breathing or body scans can help you tune into your physical and emotional state.

Pay attention to physical signs of emotional distress as well. Fatigue, changes in appetite, difficulty sleeping, or unexplained aches and pains can all indicate that you're struggling with unaddressed grief.

By becoming more attuned to your emotional and physical state, you'll be better equipped to identify when you need extra support or self-care.

The Grief Compass Technique

The Grief Compass Technique is a great method for getting through caregiver grief.

This approach helps you map out your emotions and develop personalized coping strategies.

Here's how to apply it:

1. Identify your grief patterns and triggers

Take note of situations, events, or times of day that tend to evoke strong emotions. Are there particular care tasks that leave you feeling especially sad or frustrated?

Do certain memories or milestones trigger intense feelings of loss?

Create a "grief map" by noting these patterns. This visual representation can help you anticipate and prepare for difficult moments.

2. Develop tailored coping strategies

Based on your identified patterns, create a toolkit of coping mechanisms. For moments of acute sadness, you might use deep breathing exercises or call a supportive friend.

If you're feeling overwhelmed, try breaking tasks into smaller, manageable steps.

If you experience anger, consider physical outlets like going for a walk or doing yoga.

Experiment with different strategies to find what's most effective for you. Keep your toolkit easily accessible, whether it's a list on your phone or a physical card you carry with you.

3. Find purpose amidst loss

Reflect on the values that drive your caregiving. How does this role align with your core beliefs?

Consider ways to honor your loved one's legacy, such as sharing their stories or continuing traditions they valued. Explore how your caregiving experience has changed you.

Have you developed new strengths or insights?

Finding meaning in your caregiving role can provide a sense of purpose and help you survive the grieving process. It doesn't reduce the pain of loss, but it can offer a different perspective on your experience.

4. Practice self-reflection exercises

Incorporate regular activities that promote emotional processing:

- Gratitude practice: Each day, write down three things you're grateful for, no matter how small.

- Letter writing: Write a letter to your loved one expressing your feelings. You don't need to send it—the act of writing can be cathartic.

- Values assessment: Regularly review your personal values and how they align with your caregiving role.

- Emotion tracking: Use a mood tracker app or journal to watch your emotional state over time.

By consistently engaging in these exercises, you'll develop a deeper understanding of your grief process and build resilience.

Building Your Support Network

Join a support group specifically for dementia caregivers. These groups offer a safe space to share your feelings, exchange practical advice, and connect with others who understand your experience.

Many communities offer in-person support groups, and there are numerous online options if attending in person is challenging.

Don't hesitate to lean on friends and family for support. Be specific about what you need, whether it's a listening ear, help with practical tasks, or simply some time for yourself. Many cities and towns offer respite care options for people with dementia, providing a safe and supportive environment where your loved one can be looked after for a few hours. In many cases, these services can become a regular part of the week to give both the person with dementia and their carer a much-needed break.

Accepting help strengthens your ability to provide sustainable care.

A therapist or counselor experienced in grief and caregiving issues can provide valuable coping strategies and a neutral space to process your emotions.

Look for professionals who specialize in:

- **Individual therapy**
- **Family counseling**
- **Grief counseling**

Your loved one's healthcare team can also be a valuable resource, as they can provide information about the progression of dementia and help you prepare for future changes.

Don't hesitate to ask questions or express your concerns during medical appointments.

Self-Care Strategies for Caregivers

Caring for yourself is essential for sustainable caregiving. Here are some strategies to incorporate into your routine:

Practice self-compassion: Be kind and remind yourself that you're doing the best you can in a challenging situation. Avoid self-criticism and treat yourself with the same compassion you extend to your loved one.

Seek moments of joy: While caregiving can be overwhelming, try to find small moments of happiness each day. This could be as simple as enjoying a cup of coffee in a quiet moment or sharing a laugh with your loved one.

Express your emotions creatively: Consider channeling your grief into creative outlets such as writing, painting, or music. These activities can provide a healthy way to process your feelings and create something meaningful from your experience.

Maintain your own health: Grief can take a physical toll, so prioritize your own health needs. Ensure you're getting enough sleep, eating nutritious meals, and engaging in regular physical activity. Schedule regular check-ups with your healthcare provider to watch your own well-being.

Set realistic expectations: Recognize that there will be good days and bad days. It's okay to have moments of frustration or sadness—these don't negate your love or commitment to your caregiving role.

Prioritizing Your Needs

Caregivers often focus so intently on their loved one's needs, that they neglect their own. This can lead to burnout, depression, and a diminished ability to provide quality care. Recognizing that your needs matter is the first step towards effective self-care.

To start prioritizing your needs, make a list of activities that rejuvenate you. These might include reading a book, taking a walk, or calling a friend.

Commit to incorporating at least one of these activities into your daily routine. Taking care of yourself allows you to be a better caregiver for your loved one.

Rest and Rejuvenation

Adequate rest is essential to your physical and mental health. If you're caring for someone with dementia, sleep is often disrupted or sacrificed. Here are some strategies to confirm you get the rest you need:

Establish a consistent sleep routine by going to bed and waking up at the same time each day, even on weekends. This helps regulate your body's internal clock, making it easier to fall asleep and wake up naturally.

Create a sleep-friendly bedroom. Keep it dark, quiet, and cool. Consider using blackout curtains, a white noise machine, or earplugs if needed. The ideal sleeping temperature for most people is between 60-67°F (15-19°C).

Practice relaxation techniques before bed to calm your mind, such as deep breathing exercises, progressive muscle relaxation, or gentle stretching. These activities can help reduce stress and prepare your body for sleep.

Limit screen time at least an hour before bedtime. The blue light emitted by electronic devices can interfere with your body's production of melatonin, the hormone that regulates sleep. Instead, try reading a book or listening to calming music.

Arrange respite care to allow for uninterrupted sleep. This could involve asking a family member to stay overnight occasionally or hiring a professional caregiver for nighttime shifts.

Taking breaks throughout the day can help you recharge. Even a few minutes of quiet time or a brief walk can make a significant difference in your energy levels and mood.

Setting Boundaries

Establishing and maintaining boundaries is important for your well-being and the quality of care you provide.

Here's how you can set healthy boundaries:

Learn to say no to extra responsibilities or invitations when you're already stretched thin. It's okay to decline politely and explain that you need to focus on your caregiving duties and self-care.

Communicate your limits and needs clearly to family members, friends, and healthcare providers. Be specific about what you can and cannot do, and don't be afraid to ask for help when needed.

Prioritize tasks by focusing on what's most important and letting go of less critical duties. Use a to-do list or a planner to help you organize your responsibilities and identify areas where you can delegate or simplify and set realistic expectations for yourself.

Understand that you can't do everything perfectly, and that's okay. Aim for "good enough" as opposed to perfection in your caregiving and personal tasks.

Create a personal space in your home that's just for you. This could be a corner of your bedroom, a comfortable chair by a window, or even a small outdoor area. Use this space to retreat when you need a moment of peace or to engage in activities that bring you joy.

Overcoming Common Obstacles

Even with the best intentions, caregivers often face obstacles in prioritizing self-care.

Here are some common challenges and strategies to overcome them:

Time constraints often make caregivers feel like they can't fit self-care into their busy schedules. To address this, try breaking self-care activities into smaller, manageable chunks throughout the day. Even five minutes of deep breathing or a quick stretch can make a difference.

Feeling selfish about taking time for yourself is a common struggle for caregivers. Remind yourself that self-care enables you to provide better care for your loved one.

It's not selfish to maintain your own health and well-being—it's necessary.

Financial limitations can make some self-care activities seem out of reach. Explore free or low-cost options, such as community classes, online resources, or simple activities like taking a walk in nature or practicing meditation using free apps or YouTube videos.

Lack of energy often prevents caregivers from engaging in self-care activities. Start with small, low-energy activities and gradually build up as you feel more energized. Remember that many self-care practices, like gentle stretching or deep breathing, can help increase your energy levels over time.

Difficulty leaving your loved one alone can make it challenging to engage in self-care activities outside the home. Explore in-home respite care options or activities you can do while still being present, such as listening to audiobooks or doing gentle exercises while your loved one rests.

Being Your Best Self

By acknowledging your emotions, implementing coping strategies, and seeking support, you can get through this while continuing to provide compassionate care for your loved one.

Remember that your feelings are valid, your efforts are valuable, and your well-being matters. Taking care of yourself isn't selfish—it's essential to sustain your caregiving role and maintaining your own health.

There will be difficult days, but there will also be moments of connection, love, and even joy. By honoring your grief and tending to your own needs, you're taking care of yourself and ensuring that you can be present and supportive for your loved one with dementia.

CHAPTER SUMMARY

17 Keys to Recognizing and Addressing Caregiver Grief

1. **Acknowledge the "long goodbye" nature of dementia caregiving.** Understand that grief is an ongoing process as you witness gradual changes in your loved one. This recognition helps you prepare emotionally for what you need to do to get results.

2. **Validate your feelings of anticipatory grief.** Accept that it's normal to grieve future losses while your loved one is still present. Don't judge yourself for these complex emotions.

3. **Keep a daily grief journal to track emotional patterns.** Set aside 10-15 minutes each day to write about your experiences and feelings. This practice helps you identify triggers and coping strategies.

4. **Practice mindfulness to increase emotional awareness.** Use techniques like deep breathing or body scans to tune into your physical and emotional state. This heightened awareness helps you address grief more effectively.

5. **Create a personalized "grief map" of triggers and patterns.** Note situations, events, or times that evoke strong emotions. Use this map to anticipate and prepare for challenging moments.

6. **Develop a toolkit of tailored coping strategies.** Based on your grief map, gather specific techniques for different emotional states. For acute sadness, you might use deep breathing. For anger, try a physical outlet like walking.

7. **Find purpose in your caregiving role.** Reflect on how caregiving aligns with your values. Consider ways to honor your loved one's legacy through your actions.

8. **Implement regular self-reflection exercises.** Incorporate activities like gratitude journaling, letter writing, or mood tracking. These practices help you process emotions and build resilience.

9. **Join a support group specifically for dementia caregivers.** Connect with others who understand your experience. Share feelings, exchange advice, and reduce isolation.

10. **Build a diverse support network beyond support groups.** Lean on friends, family, and professionals for different types of support. Be specific about your needs when you ask for help.

11. **Seek professional counseling focused on caregiver grief.** Consider working with a therapist experienced in grief and caregiving issues. They can provide specialized coping strategies and a neutral space for processing emotions.

12. **Practice daily self-compassion exercises.** Treat yourself with the same kindness you extend to your loved one. Acknowledge that you're doing your best in a challenging situation.

13. **Express your grief through creative outlets.** Channel your emotions into activities like writing, painting, or music. These provide healthy ways to process feelings and create meaning.

14. **Prioritize your physical health alongside emotional care.** Ensure you're getting enough sleep, eating well, and exercising regularly. Your physical well-being directly impacts your ability to cope with grief.

15. **Set realistic expectations for your grieving.** Recognize that there will be good days and bad days. Accept that grief isn't linear and that setbacks are normal.

16. **Establish a daily emotional check-in ritual.** Create a simple practice to process your emotions each day. This could be a few minutes of meditation, journaling, or a quiet walk.

17. **Use technology to maintain social connections.** Leverage video calls and messaging apps to stay in touch with your support network. Combat isolation even when you can't leave home.

Part IV – Preparing for the Future While Grieving the Present

CHAPTER 9
Planning for the Next Stage

As dementia progresses, the path becomes increasingly complex for both the person living with the condition and their caregivers. Planning for the future provides peace of mind during challenging times.

This chapter will guide you through the essential steps of preparing for the next stage of dementia care, addressing emotional, legal, and financial considerations that often arise.

Acknowledging the progression of dementia doesn't mean giving up hope.

Instead, it allows you to shift your focus from fighting against the inevitable to making the most of the time you have left. By accepting the reality of the situation, you can provide better care and support for your loved one.

Legal and Financial Considerations

While emotional preparation is more than necessary (and we've already gone well into that), addressing practical matters is equally important. Legal and financial considerations often take center stage as dementia progresses.

Planning ahead helps ensure that your loved one's wishes are respected and their affairs are in order.

Advanced Directives

Creating advanced directives is one of the most critical steps in this process.

These legal documents outline a person's wishes for end-of-life care and are especially important for those with dementia, who may eventually lose the ability to make decisions for themselves.

A **living will** specifies the types of medical treatments a person does or does not want to receive in end-of-life situations. A healthcare **power of attorney** designates someone to make healthcare decisions on behalf of the person if they become incapacitated.

These documents should be put in place in the early stages of dementia, while your loved one can still express their wishes and sign legal documents.

Financial Power of Attorney

Financial matters also need careful consideration.

A financial power of attorney designates someone to manage financial affairs on behalf of the person with dementia. This can include paying bills, managing bank accounts, filing taxes, making investment decisions, and applying for benefits.

Choosing a financial power of attorney should be done carefully, selecting someone who is trustworthy and capable of managing complex financial matters.

This person will have significant responsibility, so it's important to choose someone who has the time, skills, and integrity to handle these tasks effectively. You can, of course, also act as liaison between your loved one and the financial planner to oversee everything.

Estate Planning

Estate planning is another critical aspect of preparing for the future.

This involves deciding how assets will be distributed after death.

For those with dementia, it's important to address this early in the disease progression.

This process includes creating or updating a will, establishing trusts if necessary, and reviewing and updating beneficiary designations on retirement accounts and life insurance policies.

Working with an attorney who specializes in elder law can help ensure that all legal and financial matters are properly addressed. They can guide you through the complexities of estate planning, help you understand your options, and ensure that all documents are legally sound.

Honest Conversations

Open and honest communication is important when you plan for the next stage of dementia care. These conversations can be difficult, but they are essential for ensuring that everyone involved is on the same page and that the wishes of your loved one are respected.

Family Discussions

Bringing family members together to talk about the future can help prevent misunderstandings and conflicts down the road. Topics to address might include the progression of the disease and what to expect, caregiving responsibilities and how they will be shared, financial considerations and how expenses will be managed, and end-of-life care preferences.

Approach these conversations with empathy and understanding, recognizing that everyone may have different emotions and perspectives. It's important to create a safe space where all family members feel comfortable expressing their thoughts and concerns.

Conversations with Healthcare Professionals

Regular communication with healthcare providers is essential for planning suitable care.

Discuss the current stage of the disease and expected progression, treatment options and their potential benefits and risks, palliative care and hospice options, and when to consider transitioning to a higher level of care.

Don't hesitate to ask questions and seek clarification on any aspects of care that you don't understand. Healthcare professionals can provide valuable insights and guidance as they might better understand the complexities of dementia care.

Talking with Your Loved One

While it may be challenging, involving your loved one with dementia in discussions about their care is important, especially in the early stages of the disease.

This can include discussing their wishes for future care, reviewing and updating legal documents, and addressing any fears or concerns they may have about the future.

Approach these conversations with sensitivity and patience, allowing your loved one to express their thoughts and feelings at their own pace. Even if their ability to communicate or make decisions is limited, including them in the process as much as possible can help maintain their sense of dignity and autonomy.

The COMPASS Method: A Guide to Comprehensive Planning

To help you out with the planning process, consider implementing the "COMPASS Method"—a step-by-step guide I've made for the Comprehensive Planning of Advanced Stages of Dementia:

Current Situation Assessment

Begin by taking stock of your loved one's current health status, care needs, and financial situation. This assessment will serve as a baseline for future planning and help you identify immediate needs and potential challenges.

Don't overlook factors such as:

- The current stage of dementia and its impact on daily life
- Existing care arrangements and their effectiveness
- Financial resources available for care
- Current living situation and its suitability for future needs

Organize Documents

Gather all relevant legal, financial, and medical documents in one secure place. This organization will save time and reduce stress when these documents are needed. Important documents to collect include:

- Advanced directives and power of attorney documents
- Medical records and medication lists
- Insurance policies
- Bank statements and investment information
- Tax returns
- Property deeds and vehicle titles

Create both physical and digital copies of these documents for easy access and backup.

Meet with Professionals

Consult with an elder law attorney, financial advisor, and healthcare providers to talk about your options. These professionals can provide expert guidance tailored to your specific situation.

Prepare Legal Documents

Ensure that advanced directives, power of attorney, and estate planning documents are in order.

If these documents don't exist or are outdated, now is the time to create or update them.

Include:

- Living will
- Healthcare power of attorney
- Financial power of attorney
- Last will and testament
- Trusts (if suitable)

These documents should be reviewed and updated regularly, especially as circumstances change.

Articulate a Care Plan

Work with healthcare providers to create a comprehensive care plan that addresses current and future needs. This plan should be flexible and adaptable, as care needs will likely change.

Include:

- Current and anticipated care needs

- Medication management strategies

- Safety measures for the home

- Plans for social engagement and cognitive stimulation

- Strategies for managing behavioral symptoms

- Plans for respite care to support caregivers

Survey Care Options

Research different care options, including in-home care, assisted living, and memory care facilities. Understanding the range of options available will help you make informed decisions as care needs evolve.

While you're exploring care options, look over:

- Level of care provided

- Staff training and expertise in dementia care

- Safety features and security measures

- Activities and programs offered

- Cost and payment options

- Location and accessibility for family visits

Share with Family

Bring family members together to talk about the plan and address any concerns or questions.

Open communication can help prevent misunderstandings and conflicts down the road.

During these family discussions:

- Share the information you've gathered and the plans you've made

- Discuss roles and responsibilities for care

- Address any concerns or disagreements openly and respectfully

- Consider creating a written agreement or care plan that all family members can reference

The COMPASS Method is not a onetime event, but an ongoing process. As circumstances change and the disease progresses, be prepared to reassess and adjust your plans accordingly.

Additional Considerations

Cultural and Religious Beliefs

If your loved one has strong cultural or religious beliefs, ensure these are respected in the care plan and end-of-life decisions. This might involve incorporating specific rituals or practices into daily care routines, or ensuring that end-of-life care aligns with religious beliefs.

Respite Care

Caregiving can be exhausting, both physically and emotionally. Include plans for respite care to allow primary caregivers to rest and recharge.

This might involve arranging for in-home care services, adult day care programs, or short-term stays at residential care facilities.

Alternative Therapies

Some with dementia benefit from therapies like music or art therapy. Research these options and talk about them with healthcare providers.

These therapies can provide meaningful engagement and potentially improve quality of life.

Emergency Planning

Create an emergency plan that includes important contact information, medication lists, and instructions for care. This plan can be invaluable in crisis situations, ensuring that your loved one receives suitable care even if regular caregivers are unavailable.

Long-Term Care Insurance

If your loved one is in the early stages of dementia, explore long-term care insurance options to help cover future care costs. While it may be challenging to get coverage after a dementia diagnosis, it's worth investigating all potential options for financial support.

As we get through the challenging terrain of dementia care, the COMPASS Method serves as our guide, helping us chart a course through uncertain waters. By addressing emotional, legal, and financial considerations, we can face the future with greater confidence and peace of mind.

This involves making the most of the time we have with our loved ones, honoring their wishes, and providing the best possible care every step of the way. With careful planning and open communication, we can transform this difficult ordeal into one of deep connection, understanding, and love.

Reach out for support when you need it, whether from family, friends, support groups, or professionals. By taking proactive steps now, you can ensure that your loved one receives the best possible care while also protecting their wishes and assets.

This preparation allows you to focus on what truly matters—cherishing the moments you have together and providing compassionate care throughout the progression of dementia.

CHAPTER SUMMARY

10 Keys to Planning for the Next Stage of Dementia Care

1. **Acknowledge the progression and prepare emotionally.** Accept the reality of dementia's decline. This allows you to make informed decisions and focus on making the most of your time together.

2. **Create advanced directives early on.** Put living wills, healthcare power of attorney, and other orders in place while your loved one can still express their wishes.

3. **Designate a financial power of attorney.** Choose a trustworthy person to manage financial affairs. This ensures bills are paid and assets are properly managed as the disease progresses.

4. **Address estate planning with an elder law attorney.** Create or update wills, trusts, and beneficiary designations. This protects your loved one and ensures their wishes are respected.

5. **Have open conversations with family members.** Discuss care responsibilities, financial considerations, and end-of-life preferences. This prevents future conflicts and ensures everyone is on the same page.

6. **Maintain regular communication with healthcare providers.** Discuss disease progression, treatment options, and care transitions. This helps you make informed decisions about your loved one's care.

7. **Involve your loved one in care discussions when possible.** Include them in decision-making processes while they're able. This maintains their dignity and ensures their wishes are considered.

8. **Organize important documents in a secure location.** Gather medical records, legal papers, and financial information. This saves time and reduces stress when these documents are needed.

9. **Research care options for future needs.** Explore in-home care, assisted living, and memory care facilities. Understanding available options helps you plan for evolving care needs.

10. **Implement the COMPASS Method for comprehensive planning.** Use this step-by-step guide to assess the current situation, organize documents, meet with professionals, prepare legal papers, create a care plan, and involve family members.

CHAPTER 10
Coping with the Final Goodbye

When the final goodbye arrives, it brings a complex mix of emotions—relief, guilt, profound sadness, and even a sense of emptiness.

For John, whose father battled Alzheimer's for over a decade, the end came quietly one fall morning.

"I'd been preparing for this moment for years," he recalls. "But when it actually happened, I felt completely lost. It was like I'd been holding my breath for so long, and suddenly I didn't know how to breathe normally again."

His experience resonates with many caregivers and family members.

The intensity of emotions when a loved one finally passes can catch you off guard, even after years of anticipatory grief.

Anticipatory Grief vs. The Final Loss

The grief experienced after a loved one's passing often differs from what you've felt before. This difference can be attributed to the complex nature of anticipatory grief, which is the mourning process that occurs before the actual loss.

During this period, you may have already processed many aspects of the impending loss, leading to a unique emotional upheaval when the final loss occurs.

You might feel a sense of relief, which can then lead to guilt. This relief is a common and natural response, especially if your loved one had been suffering for an extended period.

The guilt that follows is often rooted in societal expectations of how we should feel after a loss, but it's important to recognize that feeling relief doesn't diminish your love for the person who has passed.

Or you may feel numb, as if you've used up all your grief already. This numbness can be a protective mechanism employed by your mind to shield you from overwhelming emotions. It's not uncommon for this numbness to persist for days, weeks, or even months after the loss, as your psyche gradually allows you to process the reality of the situation.

Some are surprised by the intensity of their emotions, even after years of anticipatory grief. This unexpected surge of feelings can occur because the finality of death brings a new dimension to the loss.

No matter how well-prepared you thought you were, the permanent absence of your loved one can trigger profound and intense emotional responses.

There's no "right" way to grieve. Your emotions are valid, whatever they may be.

Grief is a highly individual experience, influenced by factors such as your relationship with the deceased, your personal history, cultural background, and coping mechanisms.

What feels right for one person may not resonate with another, and that's perfectly acceptable.

Allow yourself the space and time to process these feelings without judgment. This means giving yourself permission to experience the full spectrum of emotions that may arise, whether they align with your expectations or not.

Finding Closure While Dealing with Mixed Emotions

Finding closure after losing a loved one to dementia presents unique challenges.

You may have already mourned the loss of the person you once knew, yet the finality of death brings its own distinct pain. Here are some strategies to help you work your way through this:

Acknowledge All Your Feelings

Allow yourself to experience the full range of emotions without self-judgment.

It's okay to feel relief alongside sadness, or to feel angry about the unfairness of the disease or at the words that were not spoken between you and your loved one or that you may not have been remembered.

Your feelings are a natural response to a difficult situation.

Reflect

Take time to remember not just the difficult final stages, but the good moments you shared throughout your loved one's life. Recall happy memories, inside jokes, and the unique qualities that made your loved one special.

This balanced perspective can help you process your grief more fully.

Seek Support

Connect with others who have gone through similar experiences. Support groups for those who have lost loved ones to dementia can provide valuable understanding and comfort. Alternatively, grief councilors or a religious/spiritual practitioner can give you the understanding and support you are seeking.

Sharing your story and listening to others can help you feel less alone in your grief.

Practice Self-Compassion

Be kind to yourself as you grieve.

Recognize that you did the best you could in a challenging situation.

Avoid self-criticism and treat yourself with the same compassion you'd offer a friend going through a similar loss.

Practical Matters

While dealing with emotional aspects of loss, you'll also need to attend to practical matters. These tasks can feel overwhelming, but they can also provide a sense of purpose during the early stages of grief.

Funeral or Memorial Service Planning

If you haven't pre-planned, you'll need to make decisions about the service. This is an opportunity to celebrate your loved one's life in a way that feels meaningful to you.

Dealing with Belongings

Sorting through your loved one's possessions can be emotionally challenging.

Take your time with this process and consider involving family members or close friends for support. You might find comfort in keeping some items as mementos or passing meaningful objects on to other family members.

Notifying Others

Informing friends, distant family, and organizations about the passing can be a painful task on its own.

Delegate some of this to trusted friends or family members and create a list to help confirm you don't overlook anyone important.

Moving Forward While Keeping Their Memory Alive

As time passes, you may find yourself ready to move forward in your life while still honoring your loved one's memory. This is a natural and healthy part of the grieving process.

Redefine Your Role

After being a caregiver for so long, it's important to rediscover who you are outside of that role. This might involve reconnecting with old hobbies or exploring new interests.

Give yourself permission to focus on your own needs and wants.

Maintain Connections

Stay in touch with the supportive network you built during your caregiving. These relationships can continue to provide comfort and understanding.

Don't be afraid to reach out when you need support or just want to talk.

Consider Counseling

If you're struggling to move forward, a grief counselor or therapist can provide valuable support and coping strategies. They can help you work through complex emotions and develop healthy ways to manage your grief.

Find Ways to Keep Their Spirit Alive

Incorporate aspects of your loved one's personality or values into your daily life. This could be as simple as using their favorite recipe, continuing a tradition they loved, or living by a principle that was important to them.

Allow Yourself Good Days and Bad Days

Grief isn't linear, and it's normal to have ups and downs. Allow yourself to have good days without guilt and be gentle with yourself on the difficult days. Both are part of the healing process.

The Transformative Nature of Grief

While painful, grief can also be a transformative experience.

Many report personal growth and increased empathy as a result of their own experience with grief.

Deeper Appreciation for Life

Having seen the fragility of life, you may find yourself more appreciative of small joys and meaningful connections. This newfound perspective can lead to a richer, more intentional way of living.

Increased Resilience

Getting through the challenges of caregiving and loss can build emotional strength and coping skills. You may find that you're better equipped to handle future challenges and support others going through difficult times.

Enhanced Empathy

Your experience may give you a deeper understanding of others' pain and a desire to support those going through similar situations. This increased empathy can enrich your relationships and lead to more meaningful connections.

Shift in Priorities

You may find yourself reevaluating what's truly important in life and making changes accordingly. This could lead to positive changes in your career, relationships, or personal goals.

Spiritual or Philosophical Growth

Confronting mortality often leads to deeper contemplation of life's big questions and can result in spiritual or philosophical growth. You might develop a new or deeper understanding of your beliefs and values.

Future Advancements in Dementia Care and Bereavement Support

As our understanding of dementia and grief continues to grow, new approaches to care and support are emerging. Technology plays an increasingly important role in both areas.

Virtual reality, for example, is used to help caregivers better understand the experience of living with dementia, potentially leading to more empathetic care. Online support groups and forums are providing new avenues for connection and support.

These digital communities can provide valuable support, especially for those who may not have access to in-person support groups.

Research into the neurobiology of grief is also advancing rapidly. Scientists are beginning to understand how grief affects the brain and how this knowledge might be used to develop more effective therapies.

Looking ahead, there's hope that advancements in dementia treatment could change the outlook of caregiving and loss.

While a cure remains elusive, researchers are making progress in developing therapies that could slow the progression of the disease or improve quality of life for those affected.

For those grieving the loss of a loved one to dementia, future developments may include more personalized approaches to bereavement support. This could involve tailored therapy programs based on individual grief responses, or the use of AI to provide round-the-clock emotional support.

To Honor Their Memory, We Must Embrace Life

The final goodbye to a loved one with dementia marks the end of a challenging chapter, but it also opens the door to a new chapter in your life. While the pain of loss may never completely disappear, it can evolve into a bittersweet reminder of the love you shared.

As you move forward, remember that your loved one's essence lives on through the memories you cherish, the values they instilled in you, and the ways their life touched others.

By honoring their memory and allowing yourself to heal, you can find a way to carry their love with you while embracing the possibilities that lie ahead.

The path through grief is deeply personal, but you don't have to walk it alone. Your loved one's legacy can continue to inspire and guide you as you work your way through this new phase of life.

CHAPTER SUMMARY

12 Keys to Coping with the Final Goodbye

1. **Acknowledge the complexity of your emotions.** Allow yourself to feel relief, guilt, sadness, or numbness without judgment. Your feelings are valid, whatever they may be.

2. **Reflect on the entire chapter, not just the end.** Take time to remember good moments shared throughout your loved one's life. This balanced perspective can help you process your grief more fully.

3. **Seek support from others who understand.** Connect with support groups for those who have lost loved ones to dementia. Sharing your story and listening to others can help you feel less alone.

4. **Practice self-compassion as you grieve.** Be kind to yourself and recognize that you did your best in a challenging situation. Avoid self-criticism and treat yourself with the same compassion you'd offer a friend.

5. **Create personal rituals for remembrance.** Establish rituals that help you feel connected to your loved one's memory. These can provide comfort and a sense of ongoing connection.

6. **Share your loved one's life story.** Write down or record their experiences, including their struggle with dementia. This preserves their memory and can educate others about the disease.

7. **Continue their passions or support their causes.** Take up a hobby they loved or volunteer for an organization they supported. This keeps their legacy alive through your actions.

8. **Establish a lasting memorial.** Create a tribute that aligns with their values and interests. This could be as simple as planting a tree or as involved as setting up a charity.

9. **Participate in dementia awareness and advocacy.** Channel your experience into helping others and pushing for better care and research. Your firsthand knowledge is invaluable.

10. **Plan a meaningful funeral or memorial service.** Celebrate your loved one's life in a way that reflects their personality and interests. This can provide closure and honor their memory.

11. **Seek professional help for legal and financial matters.** Don't hesitate to consult an attorney or financial advisor. They can guide you through necessary processes and confirm everything is handled properly.

12. **Take your time sorting through belongings.** This process can be emotionally challenging. Consider keeping some items as mementos or passing meaningful objects to family members.

13. **Delegate the task of notifying others.** Ask trusted friends or family members to help inform others about the passing. Create a list to confirm you don't overlook anyone important.

14. **Redefine your role beyond caregiving.** Rediscover who you are outside of caregiving. Give yourself permission to focus on your own needs and interests.

15. **Maintain connections with your support network.** Stay in touch with those who supported you during your caregiving. Don't be afraid to reach out when you need support.

16. **Give thought to keeping your loved one's legacy into your life.** Find ways to keep their spirit alive in your daily routines. This could be using their favorite recipe or living by a principle they valued.

17. **Allow yourself both good days and bad days.** Recognize that grief isn't linear. Be gentle with yourself on difficult days and allow yourself to enjoy good moments without guilt.

18. **Consider the transformative potential of grief.** Be open to personal growth and increased empathy that can result from your experience. This can lead to a richer, more intentional way of living.

19. **Honor their memory by embracing life.** Carry their love with you as you move forward. Your loved one's legacy can continue to inspire and guide you in this new phase of life.

Part V - Supporting Others

CHAPTER 11

Helping Family Members Cope

When dementia affects a loved one, the entire family feels the impact.

Each member processes the gradual loss differently, creating a complex web of emotions and challenges.

This chapter explores how families can weather these changes together, fostering understanding, open communication, and shared responsibility.

The Ripple Effect on Family Dynamics

As we've discussed, a dementia diagnosis changes the entire family systems. As the condition progresses, roles shift, relationships evolve, and everyone must adapt to a new reality.

Understanding typical responses helps create a more supportive environment for all involved, as well as aids in the formulation of methods to help each member of the family cope with these varied experiences of grief.

Sibling Responses

Your brothers and sisters often find themselves in unfamiliar territory when a parent develops dementia. Long-standing sibling dynamics may intensify or completely transform under the stress of caregiving.

Common reactions include:

The Primary Caregiver: Usually steps forward to manage most care responsibilities, potentially leading to burnout and resentment from others.

The Long-Distance Sibling: If there's a sibling that lives across the country, this can cause tension with those more actively engaged in daily care on both fronts. Feelings of guilt or resentment from either party.

The Reluctant Acceptor: There are those who struggle to accept the extent of their parent's decline, creating conflicts over care decisions.

The Mediator: Those who try to balance everyone's needs and ensure all voices are heard in family discussions. Sometimes, these are the fastest to experience burnout due to their attempts to hold it all together.

Younger Family Members

Children and teenagers often struggle to understand the changes in their loved one.

This difficulty in comprehension stems from their limited life experience and still-developing cognitive abilities, which can make it challenging for them to grasp the complexities of dementia or other age-related conditions. This could be particularly apparent, in the case when a loved one has early onset dementia.

The changes they observe in their loved one may seem sudden or inexplicable, leading to confusion and emotional distress. They may experience a range of emotions, from confusion and fear to sadness and anger, which can be intense and overwhelming for young family members, as they grapple with the reality of their loved one's declining health.

Confusion may arise from not fully understanding the nature of the condition, while fear can be triggered by the unpredictability of the situation or concerns about their own future.

Sadness is a natural response to witnessing the deterioration of a beloved family member, and anger might manifest as frustration with the situation or even resentment towards the affected person for changing.

Grandchildren might feel a profound sense of loss as their relationship with a grandparent changes. This sense of loss can be particularly acute for grandchildren who have before enjoyed a close bond with their grandparent.

As the grandparent's cognitive abilities decline, shared activities, conversations, and traditions that once defined their relationship may become difficult or impossible to maintain. This shift can leave grandchildren feeling bereft of the emotional support and guidance they before received from their grandparent.

It's important to be there for them to lean on, especially now more than ever.

Extended Family

Aunts, uncles, and cousins may feel uncertain about their role in the caregiving process.

This uncertainty can stem from various factors, including geographical distance, pre-existing family dynamics, or a lack of clear communication about caregiving needs. They might struggle to determine how much involvement is suitable or expected of them, especially if they are not part of the immediate caregiving circle. This uncertainty can lead to increased involvement for some and withdrawal for others.

Those who respond with increased involvement may feel compelled to offer more support, potentially rearranging their own lives to accommodate caregiving responsibilities. This can manifest as more frequent visits, financial contributions, or taking on specific caregiving tasks. On the other hand, family members who withdraw might do so because of feelings of helplessness, fear of interfering, or their own emotional struggles with the situation.

Fostering Open Communication

Clear, honest communication forms the foundation for helping family members cope with dementia.

Here are strategies to promote better family dialogue:

Regular Family Meetings

Schedule consistent times for all involved family members to connect, either in person or virtually. These meetings provide a forum to discuss care plans, share concerns, and make decisions collaboratively.

Set an agenda beforehand and confirm everyone has a chance to speak.

Create a Safe Space for Feelings

Encourage all family members to express their emotions without fear of judgment.

Acknowledge that there's no "correct" way to feel about the situation. You might say, "I know this is hard for everyone. Let's try to be open about how we're feeling, even if it's difficult."

Use "I" Statements

When discussing challenges or frustrations, frame your thoughts using "I" statements. For example, instead of saying, "You never help with Dad," try, "I feel overwhelmed and could use more support." This approach reduces defensiveness and promotes understanding.

Consider Professional Help

If conflicts continue or communication breaks down, a family therapist or mediator specializing in eldercare issues can facilitate productive discussions. They can provide neutral ground and tools for working through complex family dynamics.

Leverage Technology

Set up a group chat or use caregiving apps to keep everyone informed and involved, even from a distance. This ensures that all family members have access to the same information and can contribute to decision-making.

A Family Approach to Caregiving

Distributing caregiving responsibilities among family members prevents burnout and ensures comprehensive care for the person with dementia.

Here's how to encourage shared responsibility:

Play to Individual Strengths

Recognize that each family member brings unique skills and abilities to the table. Some excel at hands-on care, while others are better suited for managing finances or coordinating medical appointments.

Encourage family members to take on roles that align with their strengths and comfort levels. For example, your tech-savvy nephew might set up a medication reminder system, while your nurturing sister takes on more personal care tasks.

Who does what can also depend on how your loved one reacts to different family members for whatever reason. Be open to reassessing roles as needs change throughout the progression of the disease.

Create a Shared Care Calendar

Use online tools to create a calendar where family members can sign up for specific tasks or time slots. This visual representation helps everyone see what needs to be done and who's responsible.

Include not just direct care tasks, and:

- Grocery shopping and meal preparation

- House cleaning and maintenance

- Medication management

- Transportation to appointments

- Social visits and activities

Regular updates keep everyone in the loop, even those who can't be there in person every day. Try out different apps or platforms to find one that works best for your family's needs and tech comfort levels.

Rotate Demanding Tasks

To prevent resentment and burnout, consider rotating more challenging responsibilities among capable family members. This might mean taking turns with overnight care or switching who handles the most stressful appointments.

Be flexible with the rotation schedule. Life happens, and sometimes we all do need to swap shifts or take a break.

Maintain open communication about needs and limitations.

Remember that not all tasks need to be rotated.

If someone genuinely enjoys or excels at a particular aspect of care, it's okay for that to be their consistent role.

Value Long-Distance Contributions

Family members who live far away can still make meaningful contributions.

They might provide financial support, manage paperwork, or offer emotional support to the primary caregiver.

Long-distance caregivers often feel guilty about not being there in person. Validate their efforts, no matter how small they may seem.

A weekly video call to provide companionship or handling online bill payments are valuable contributions. Encourage long-distance family members to visit when possible, both to spend time with the person with dementia and to give local caregivers a break.

Respect Individual Circumstances

Understand that not everyone can contribute equally because of their own life situations. Some family members may have young children, demanding careers, or health issues that limit their availability.

Pushing too hard can lead to resentment or finish withdrawal.

Instead, focus on finding ways for everyone to contribute in a way that fits their current situation. Maybe the busy working mom can't provide daily care, but she can handle weekly grocery deliveries or take the lead on researching care options.

Be willing to reassess and adjust expectations as family circumstances change.

Involving Younger Family Members

Children and teenagers often have a unique ability to connect with their loved one, even as dementia progresses.

Here are age-appropriate ways to involve younger family members:

For Children (Ages 5-12)

Encourage kids to create artwork or cards for their loved one. This creative outlet allows them to express their feelings and maintain a connection.

Involve them in simple, safe tasks like setting the table or reading aloud, which can help children feel useful and included in the caregiving process.

Help them understand dementia through age-appropriate books and resources. Answer their questions honestly, but in terms they can grasp. You might say, "Grandpa's brain is changing, which makes it hard for him to remember things sometimes. But he still loves you very much."

For Teenagers (Ages 13-18)

Teach teens how to assist with basic care tasks under supervision, which can include helping with meals or accompanying their loved one on short walks.

This preserves family history and provides a meaningful way for teens to connect with their loved one. Involve them in planning activities or outings suitable for the person with dementia. This responsibility helps teens feel valued and teaches them about adapting to changing needs.

For Young Adults

Include young adult family members in care planning discussions. Their perspective can be valuable, and it prepares them for potential future caregiving roles.

Encourage them to spend one-on-one time with their loved one, focusing on activities they can still enjoy together.

Teach them about managing medications or using assistive technologies. This practical knowledge builds their confidence and ability to contribute to care.

Coping Strategies for Different Family Members

Each family member may need different types of support to cope with the ongoing loss associated with dementia.

Here are tailored strategies for various family roles:

For Adult Children

Join a support group specifically for adult children of parents with dementia.

Sharing experiences with others in similar situations can provide comfort and practical advice.

You can try seeking therapy, as an individual or as a group, to process complex emotions and family dynamics. A therapist can help you vent feelings of grief, guilt, or anger that often accompany caregiving.

For Spouses

Connect with other spouses of dementia patients for peer support.

Local support groups or online forums can provide a sense of community and understanding.

Maintain some aspects of your relationship that don't revolve around caregiving. This might include watching favorite shows together or continuing shared hobbies when possible. Plan for the future, including legal and financial considerations. While difficult, addressing these issues early can reduce stress later.

For Siblings

Have open discussions about shared caregiving responsibilities. Be honest about what each sibling can realistically contribute, considering factors like geographic location, work commitments, and personal strengths.

Acknowledge and work through long-standing sibling dynamics that may affect caregiving as old rivalries or resentments can resurface under stress, so addressing them directly is essential. It's also important to support each other's self-care efforts. Recognize when a sibling needs a break and offer to step in or arrange respite care.

Remember that you're all on the same team, even if you don't always agree on every decision.

For Grandchildren

Provide age-appropriate education about dementia.

Help grandchildren understand the changes they're seeing in their grandparent without overwhelming them with medical details.

Encourage them to maintain a relationship with their grandparent through activities they can still enjoy together. This might include looking at photo albums, listening to music, or simple crafts.

Offer emotional support and opportunities for grandchildren to express their feelings about the changes they observe. Create a safe space for them to ask questions and share concerns. Validate their emotions and reassure them that it's okay to feel sad, confused, or even angry sometimes.

Move Forward Together

Helping family members cope with the gradual loss of a loved one to dementia is undoubtedly challenging. It will test your patience, stretch your resources, and sometimes push you to your limits.

But it can also reveal strengths you never knew you had, deepen family bonds, and provide moments of profound connection and love.

As you work your way along this path, be gentle with yourself and your family members. You're all doing the best you can in a difficult situation.

Celebrate victories, forgive imperfections, and remember that your presence and care make a difference, even on the hardest days.

By fostering open communication, encouraging shared responsibilities, and involving all family members in age-appropriate ways, you can create a support network that benefits both the person with dementia and each other.

There's no perfect way to get through this unscathed, but by working together and supporting one another, families can find strength, resilience, and even moments of joy amidst the challenges of dementia caregiving.

CHAPTER SUMMARY

17 Keys to Helping Family Members Cope with Dementia

1. **Foster open communication among all family members.** Schedule regular family meetings to talk about care plans and concerns. Create a safe space for everyone to express their feelings without judgment.

2. **Distribute caregiving responsibilities based on personal strengths.** Recognize that each family member has different skills and abilities. Encourage them to take on roles that align with their strengths and comfort levels.

3. **Create a shared care calendar for task management.** Use online tools to create a calendar where family members can sign up for specific tasks or time slots. Include both direct care and support tasks.

4. **Rotate demanding tasks to prevent caregiver burnout.** Consider taking turns with challenging responsibilities like overnight care. Be flexible with the rotation schedule to accommodate changing needs.

5. **Acknowledge and value long-distance family contributions.** Recognize that family members who live far away can still contribute through financial support, managing paperwork, or providing emotional support.

6. **Respect personal circumstances and limitations of family members.** Understand that not everyone can contribute equally because of their own life situations. Focus

on finding ways for everyone to help that fit their current circumstances.

7. **Involve children in age-appropriate caregiving activities.** Encourage kids to create artwork or help with simple tasks. This helps them feel included and maintains their connection with their loved one.

8. **Engage teenagers in more substantial care responsibilities.** Teach teens how to assist with basic care tasks under supervision. Involve them in planning activities suitable for the person with dementia.

9. **Include young adults in care planning discussions.** Encourage them to spend one-on-one time with their loved one. Teach them about managing medications or using assistive technologies.

10. **Connect adult children with support groups and resources.** Encourage them to join support groups specifically for adult children of parents with dementia. Suggest therapy to process complex emotions.

11. **Help spouses maintain aspects of their relationship.** Encourage them to continue shared hobbies when possible. Connect them with peer support from other spouses of those with dementia.

12. **Address long-standing sibling dynamics affecting caregiving.** Have open discussions about shared responsibilities among siblings. Support each other's self-care efforts and offer to step in when a sibling needs a break.

13. **Provide age-appropriate education about dementia for grandchildren.** Help them understand the changes they're seeing without overwhelming them. Offer emotional support and opportunities to express their feelings.

14. **Focus on creating meaningful connections in the present.** Engage in activities that bring joy in the moment, even if they're different from past interactions. Embrace simple pleasures like holding hands or listening to music together.

15. **Utilize technology to keep all family members involved.** Set up group chats or use caregiving apps to keep everyone informed. This ensures all family members have access to the same information and can contribute to decision-making.

16. **Consider professional mediation for unresolved family conflicts.** If communication breaks down, a family therapist or mediator specializing in eldercare issues can facilitate productive discussions.

17. **Celebrate small victories and forgive imperfections.** Remember that you're all doing your best in a difficult situation. Acknowledge the challenges and recognize moments of connection and love.

CHAPTER 12

Empowering Friends to Provide Support

"Friendship is born at that moment when one person says to another, 'What! You too? I thought I was the only one.'"
C.S. Lewis

The support of friends can make a world of difference when caring for someone with dementia.

Many *do* want to help but feel unsure about how to offer meaningful assistance, or cannot offer effective support, simply because they don't understand.

By educating friends about dementia and providing specific ways they can contribute, you'll create a strong network of support for both you and your loved one.

Understanding Dementia: A Guide for Friends

Before friends can offer effective support, they need to grasp the basics of dementia.

Here's a concise explanation you can share:

Dementia describes a decline in mental ability severe enough to interfere with daily life.

Alzheimer's disease causes 60-80% of dementia cases.

Dementia affects memory, thinking, behavior, and emotions.

Symptoms gradually worsen over time.

Key points to emphasize:

- Dementia is *not* a normal part of aging

- It affects each person differently

- The person with dementia is still the same person, even as their abilities and personality change

Practical Ways Friends Can Help

Be Present

Sometimes the most valuable support is simply being there. Encourage friends to visit, call, or send messages regularly. Let them know that their presence alone can provide comfort and connection.

Listen Without Judgment

Provide a safe space for caregivers to express their feelings, fears, and frustrations.

Active, empathetic listening allows caregivers to process their emotions and feel understood.

Offer Tangible Assistance

Suggest specific tasks friends can do to lighten the load:

- Prepare and deliver meals

- Run errands like grocery shopping or picking up prescriptions

- Help with household chores like laundry, dishes, or yard work

- Provide respite care to allow the primary caregiver a break

Stay Connected

Maintain friendships by including the person with dementia and their caregiver in social activities when possible.

Adapt gatherings to accommodate their needs and abilities.

Learn More

Encourage friends to educate themselves about dementia through reputable sources like the Alzheimer's Association or local support groups. The more they understand, the better equipped they'll be to offer meaningful support.

Provide Emotional Support

A hug, a kind word, or simply sitting together in silence can be incredibly comforting.

Small gestures of care and compassion make a big difference.

Remember Special Occasions

Continue to acknowledge birthdays, anniversaries, and holidays. These gestures mean a lot to both the person with dementia and their caregiver, helping them feel remembered and valued.

Encourage Self-Care

Support the caregiver in taking time for themselves. Offer to help make that possible by providing respite care or assisting with tasks that free up the caregiver's time.

Foster Inclusion

Include the person with dementia in conversations and activities as much as possible. Adapt interactions to their current abilities, focusing on what they can still do rather than what they've lost.

Empowering Friends: A Step-by-Step Approach

Initiate the Conversation

Reach out to close friends and explain your situation. Be honest about the challenges you're facing and the support you need. Many friends want to help but don't know how to start the conversation themselves.

Educate

Share resources about dementia, such as brochures from the Alzheimer's Association or reputable websites. Offer to answer questions they might have.

Knowledge empowers friends to interact more confidently with your loved one.

Be Specific

Instead of saying "I'll let you know if I need anything," provide concrete ways friends can help.

For example, "Could you bring a meal once a week?" or "Would you be able to stay with my mother for two hours on Saturday so I can run errands?" Specific requests make it easier for friends to say yes and follow through.

Create a Support Schedule

Use online tools like care calendars to organize help from multiple friends.

This prevents overlap and confirms consistent support. It also allows friends to choose tasks that fit their schedules and comfort levels.

Encourage Interaction

Invite friends to spend time with the person who has dementia. Provide tips on communication and suggest activities they can do together, which could include looking at photo albums, listening to music, or going for short walks.

Express Gratitude

Regularly thank friends for their support.

This encouragement helps them feel valued and more likely to continue helping.

A simple thank-you note, or phone call, goes a long way in showing appreciation.

Update Regularly

Keep friends informed about changes in your loved one's condition and any new needs that arise. Regular updates help friends understand how to best support you as the situation advances.

Facilitate Group Support

Think about organizing a small gathering of friends to talk about how they can work together to provide support. This encourages teamwork and allows friends to coordinate their efforts.

Encourage Self-Care

Remind friends that supporting someone with dementia can be emotionally challenging.

Encourage them to take care of their own well-being too. This might include setting boundaries or taking breaks when needed.

Be Open to Different Forms of Support

Remember that friends may offer support in various ways. Some may excel at practical tasks, while others provide emotional support. Appreciate all forms of help, recognizing that diversity in support strengthens your overall network.

Creating a Dementia Communication Guide

To further empower friends, consider creating a simple guide with tips on how to talk effectively with someone who has dementia.

Include suggestions like:

- Speak slowly and clearly

- Use simple sentences and avoid complex language

- Allow them plenty of extra time for responses

- Avoid arguing or correcting mistakes

- Use visual cues or gestures to support verbal communication

- Focus on feelings rather than facts

- Maintain a calm and reassuring demeanor

This guide gives friends concrete tools to interact more confidently with your loved one, reducing anxiety and promoting positive interactions.

To Empower Friends, Approach with Communication and Gratitude

Empowering friends to provide support needs clear communication, education, and ongoing appreciation. By helping friends understand dementia and providing specific ways they can help, you create a strong network of care.

This network aids in practical matters and provides emotional sustenance during a challenging ordeal.

Every act of support, no matter how small, can make a significant difference. Working together, friends can help lighten the load, provide moments of joy, and confirm that both you and your loved one with dementia feel supported throughout this experience.

CHAPTER SUMMARY

14 Keys to Empowering Friends to Support Dementia Care

1. **Educate friends about dementia basics.** Provide a concise explanation of what dementia is and how it affects daily life. Emphasize that it's not a normal part of aging and affects each person differently.

2. **Be specific when you're asking for help.** Remember: instead of general requests, provide concrete tasks friends can do. This makes it easier for them to say yes and follow through.

3. **Create a support schedule using online tools.** Use care calendars to organize help from multiple friends. This prevents overlap and ensures consistent support.

4. **Encourage friends to maintain social connections.** Invite friends to include your loved one in social activities when possible. Adapt gatherings to accommodate their needs and abilities.

5. **Provide a "Dementia Communication Guide" for friends.** Create a simple guide with tips on how to effectively talk with someone who has dementia. Include practical suggestions for positive interactions.

6. **Use technology for coordination and updates.** Set up a group chat or email list to keep friends informed about your loved one's condition and new needs. This streamlines communication effectively.

7. **Encourage friends to offer emotional support.** Remind friends that sometimes just being present and listening

without judgment is incredibly valuable. Small gestures of care make a big difference.

8. **Suggest practical ways friends can help.** Provide a list of specific tasks like preparing meals, running errands, or doing household chores. Be clear about what would be most helpful to you.

9. **Emphasize patience and flexibility.** Remind friends that those with dementia have good days and bad days. Encourage them to be understanding and adaptable.

10. **Create opportunities for respite care.** Ask friends to provide short periods of care to allow you breaks. This helps prevent caregiver burnout and maintains your well-being.

11. **Encourage friends to continue acknowledging special occasions.** Ask friends to remember birthdays, anniversaries, and holidays. These gestures mean a lot to both you and your loved one with dementia.

12. **Foster inclusion in conversations and activities.** Guide friends on how to include your loved one in interactions, focusing on their current abilities rather than limitations.

13. **Express gratitude regularly for support received.** Thank friends often for their help. This encouragement helps them feel valued and more likely to continue supporting you.

14. **Be open to different forms of support from friends.** Recognize that friends may offer help in various ways. Appreciate all forms of assistance, whether practical or emotional.

Part VI – Moving Forward with Love and Resilience

CHAPTER 13
Life After Loss

When a loved one with dementia passes away, you'll likely find yourself grieving two distinct losses. First, there's the gradual loss of the person you once knew, which occurred throughout the disease progression.

Second, there's the physical loss of your loved one and the end of your caregiving role.

This dual nature of loss can complicate the grieving process, as you may feel you've already done much of your grieving, yet still experience intense emotions after your loved one's death.

In the aftermath of loss, you may experience a range of emotions.

Feeling relief from the demands of caregiving and witnessing your loved one's decline is common and normal. You might also feel guilt, either for experiencing relief or for perceived shortcomings in your caregiving.

Confusion about how to grieve someone who may have seemed "already gone" in many ways, is also typical. Many caregivers report a profound sense of emptiness, both for the person who died and for their own role and identity as a caregiver. Some experience emotional numbness as a temporary way of coping with overwhelming feelings.

All of these reactions are valid parts of the grieving process.

The Immediate Aftermath

The days and weeks following the loss of a loved one to dementia can feel overwhelming.

Here are some strategies to help you through this initial period:

Allow yourself to fully experience your emotions. There's no need to suppress or rush your feelings.

Crying, anger, and numbness are all valid parts of your grieving process.

Give yourself permission to feel whatever comes up without judgment.

Reach out to the support network you've been building all this time.

Family, friends, or support groups can provide invaluable comfort during this time.

Don't hesitate to ask for help with practical matters or simply for a listening ear.

Sharing your feelings with others who understand can be incredibly comforting.

Prioritize your physical health. Grief can take a toll on your body, so it's important to maintain regular sleep patterns, eat nutritious meals, and engage in gentle exercise.

Even small acts of self-care can make a significant difference in your ability to cope with the emotional challenges you're facing.

Handle practical matters gradually. While there are necessary tasks to be done, such as arranging the funeral or dealing with legal matters, don't feel pressured to handle everything at once.

Focus on what needs immediate attention and delegate tasks when possible.

Give yourself time and space to process your loss.

Creating a meaningful memorial can be a healing process, if you haven't done so already.

Plan a service or tribute that reflects your loved one's life and values (more on this in the next chapter).

Honor their life before dementia as well as the strength they showed throughout their illness. This can be a powerful way to celebrate their memory and begin the healing process.

Healing

Healing from the loss of a loved one to dementia takes time, with ups and downs along the way.

Here are some strategies to support your healing:

Acknowledge the full spectrum of your loss. You're grieving the person who died and the dreams and future you had imagined with them.

Many caregivers also mourn the loss of their caregiving role, which, despite its challenges, gave their days' structure and purpose.

Practice self-compassion. Be kind to yourself as you make your way through this new reality.

Avoid self-criticism or comparing your grief to others.

Remember that healing takes time, and there's no set timeline for when you should feel "better."

If you're struggling to cope or feeling stuck in your grief, **seek help from a grief counselor or therapist**. They can provide tools and strategies tailored to your specific situation, helping you through the pain that inevitably comes with this type of loss.

Connecting with others who have experienced similar losses can be incredibly validating and healing. Join a support group for those who have lost loved ones to dementia. Sharing your experiences with others who have walked a similar path can provide comfort and practical coping strategies.

Rediscovering Your Identity and Purpose

Caring for someone with dementia often becomes all-encompassing, and many caregivers find themselves at a loss when that role ends. Rediscovering who you are outside of caregiving is an important part of healing and moving forward.

Take time to reconnect with the things that were important to you before caregiving took center stage.

Reflect on the activities that brought you joy and the values that guided your life, and use these reflections as a starting point for exploring new or renewed pursuits.

When it comes to making changes in your life, start small and don't pressure yourself to make big life changes immediately. Begin with manageable steps, such as taking a class in a subject that interests you, volunteering for a cause you care about, or reconnecting with old friends.

These small actions can help you gradually rebuild your purpose and identity.

After years of focusing on someone else's needs, it's time to prioritize your own well-being. Schedule check-ups, address any health concerns you've been neglecting, and establish routines that support your physical and mental health.

Consider how you might use your caregiving experience in new ways. Some former caregivers find purpose in giving advice to new caregivers, advocating for better dementia care and support, or writing about their experiences to help others.

Your unique insights and experiences can be invaluable to others facing similar challenges.

Throughout this process of rediscovery, be gentle with yourself. It's normal to have days where you feel lost or unsure—these are natural parts of the healing process.

Allow yourself the time and space to explore and adjust to your new circumstances.

Cherishing Their Legacy

As you move forward, it's possible to build a fulfilling life while still honoring your loved one's memory.

Here are some ways to achieve this balance:

Integrate their legacy into your life by thinking about the values, lessons, or qualities your loved one embodied. Carry these forward in your own life. This might involve adopting a cause they cared about, or embodying a quality they exemplified, such as kindness or resilience.

Create new traditions that honor your loved one while also reflecting your current life. This could be an annual gathering with family and friends to share memories, or a personal ritual like visiting a favorite place on their birthday.

These new traditions can help you maintain a connection to your loved one while also acknowledging the changes in your life.

Remember that experiencing happiness and moving forward with your life doesn't reduce your love for the person you lost. They would likely want you to find joy and fulfillment, so allow yourself to embrace new experiences and opportunities for happiness as they arise.

Maintain connections with family and friends who were part of your caregiving experience and be open to forming new relationships. Your shared history is important, but new connections can also enrich your life and provide fresh perspectives.

Reflect on what your loved one would have wanted for you.

It's a heartwarming fact that, even in later stages during moments of lucidity, many who struggle with dementia express a desire for their family members to live full, happy lives after they're gone. Honoring them by striving to do just that can be a powerful way to carry their memory forward.

Exercises for Healing and Growth

Journaling can be a powerful tool for processing your emotions and tracking your healing process.

Set aside time each day to write about your feelings, memories, and experiences to help you gain clarity and perspective on your grief.

Planning a month of small, daily self-care activities can help you prioritize your well-being. This could include taking a walk, reading a book, or calling a friend. Having these activities planned out in advance can give you something to look forward to each day.

Such projects can help you feel connected to your loved one while also contributing something positive to the world.

A Continuing Bond of Love and Memory

The end of your loved one's suffering with dementia marks the beginning of a new chapter in your own life.

While the pain of loss may never completely fade, healing, rediscovering your sense of self, and building a meaningful future that honors your loved one's memory are all possible.

Remember that this process is deeply personal, and there's no "right" way to grieve or move forward. Your loved one's legacy lives on through you, in the love you shared, the memories you cherish, and the life you continue to live.

Be gentle with yourself, remain open to new experiences, and always be mindful of the enduring connection and love you shared with your loved one. It doesn't end with their passing—it continues to shape and enrich your life in countless ways.

Some days will be harder than others, and that's okay.

What matters is that you continue to move forward, one step at a time, honoring your loved one's memory while also embracing the possibilities that lie ahead.

Your experience as a caregiver has likely given you strength, compassion, and resilience that you may not have realized you possessed. These qualities can serve you well as you build your new life. Use these strengths to enrich your life and the lives of others.

Finally, give yourself permission to find joy and purpose in your life again.

Doing so doesn't mean you're forgetting your loved one or that your love for them has diminished. Instead, it's a testament to the richness of the life you shared and the strength they helped instill in you. Your loved one's greatest legacy may be the love and resilience they fostered in you—carry that forward with pride and gratitude.

CHAPTER SUMMARY

24 Keys to Healing After Losing a Loved One to Dementia

1. **Allow yourself to experience all emotions fully.** Don't suppress your feelings.

   Give yourself permission to cry, be angry, or feel numb.

2. **Recognize the unique nature of dementia-related grief.** Remember that you may have experienced anticipatory grief and are now compounding that as you face dual loss.

3. **Lean on your support system for help.** Reach out to family, friends, or support groups.

   Don't hesitate to ask for assistance with practical matters or emotional support.

4. **Prioritize your physical health during grief.** Maintain regular sleep patterns, eat nutritious meals, and engage in gentle exercise.

   Small acts of self-care can significantly impact your ability to cope.

5. **Handle practical matters gradually after the loss.** Focus on immediate necessities and delegate tasks when possible.

   Don't pressure yourself to handle everything at once.

6. **Create a meaningful memorial for your loved one.** Plan a service or tribute that reflects their life and values, honoring both their pre-dementia self and their current state with the disease.

7. **Acknowledge the full spectrum of your loss.** Recognize that you're grieving both the person who died and the dreams you had for your shared future.

8. **Practice self-compassion throughout your healing.** Be kind to yourself as you make your way through this new reality.

   Avoid self-criticism or comparing your grief to others.

9. **Find ways to honor your loved one's memory.** Continue their traditions, or support dementia research in their name.

10. **Connect with others who understand dementia loss.** Join a support group for those who have lost loved ones to dementia.

    Sharing experiences can be validating and healing.

11. **Reflect on your values and interests post-caregiving.** Take time to reconnect with activities and principles that were important to you before caregiving took center stage.

12. **Start small when making life changes.** Begin with manageable steps like taking a class, volunteering, or reconnecting with old friends.

13. **Prioritize your own well-being after years of caregiving.** Schedule check-ups, address neglected health concerns, and establish routines that support your physical and mental health.

14. **Explore new roles that use your caregiving experience.** Consider mentoring new caregivers, advocating for better dementia care, or sharing your story to help others.

15. **Integrate your loved one's legacy into your life.** Carry forward their values, lessons, or qualities they embodied in your own life and actions.

16. **Create new traditions that honor their memory.** Establish rituals that reflect both your loved one's importance and your current life circumstances.

17. **Allow yourself to experience joy without guilt.** Remember that finding happiness doesn't reduce your love for the person you lost.

18. **Maintain connections while being open to new relationships.** Stay in touch with those who shared your caregiving experience, and be open to forming new connections.

19. **Consider what your loved one would have wanted for you.** Reflect on their wishes for your future and strive to honor them by living a full life.

20. **Use journaling to process your emotions.** Set aside time each day to write about your feelings, memories, and experiences.

21. **Practice daily gratitude to shift focus.** Write down three things you're grateful for each day to cultivate a more positive outlook.

22. **Plan a month of small, daily self-care activities.** Give yourself something to look forward to each day, like taking a walk or reading a book.

23. **Start a legacy project to honor your loved one.** Channel your grief into a meaningful project, like planting a garden or creating a photo album.

24. **Embrace the ongoing nature of your connection.** Recognize that your bond with your loved one continues beyond their death, shaping your life in new ways.

CHAPTER 14
Keeping Their Memory Alive

Remembering and honoring our loved ones fulfills a basic human need. It helps us process our grief, find meaning in our experiences, and maintain a connection to those we've lost or are losing.

The loss of a loved one to dementia profoundly changes your life. After providing care and support through their struggle, you now face the challenge of honoring their memory and continuing their legacy while also reconnecting with yourself.

This chapter explores meaningful ways to remember your loved one, ensuring their impact endures long after they've gone.

Rituals and Traditions

Creating and maintaining rituals and traditions provides comfort, connection, and continuity as you endure life without your loved one. You could try having an annual remembrance day on their birthday or the anniversary of their passing. Gather family and friends to share stories, prepare their favorite meal, or visit a place that held special meaning.

A memory box or album serves as a tangible collection of mementos, photographs, and keepsakes representing your loved one's life. This treasure trove of memories allows you to revisit cherished moments and share their story with future generations.

Continuing your loved one's passions keeps their spirit alive in everyday life. If they enjoyed gardening, tend to their plants or start your own garden.

Learn to play their favorite instrument or volunteer for causes they supported.

These activities honor their memory and help you feel connected to them.

Incorporating elements of remembrance into existing holiday celebrations creates new traditions infused with their presence. Hang a special ornament on the Christmas tree, set a place for them at the Thanksgiving table, or light a candle in their memory during religious observances.

Creating a memory quilt or pillow using pieces of their clothing provides a comforting physical reminder of their presence. The tactile nature of these items can be especially soothing during difficult moments.

These are just some examples.

You'll find that there are so many ways to celebrate who they were and keep them alive in your heart.

Creative Expressions of Remembrance

Beyond traditional rituals, many creative ways exist to celebrate your loved one's life and keep their memory vibrant.

A memory garden serves as a living tribute, providing a peaceful place for reflection and remembrance. Choose plants and flowers that hold special meaning for your loved one or represent aspects of their personality. As you tend to the garden, you nurture their memory and create a beautiful space for contemplation.

If your loved one was passionate about education or a particular cause, establishing a scholarship or donation fund in their name confirms their legacy continues to make a positive impact. This lasting tribute honors their memory and helps others pursue their dreams or supports important research.

Channeling your emotions into artistic expression offers a therapeutic outlet while creating a lasting tribute. Paint a portrait or landscape that reminds you of them, capturing their essence or a special place you shared. Write poetry or songs that express your feelings or tell their story.

Craft jewelry incorporating their birthstone or favorite colors, creating a wearable reminder of their presence in your life. Memory stones offer a unique way to honor your loved one. Paint or engrave small stones with words, dates, or images representing their life and impact. Keep these in a special place at home or distribute them to family members as keepsakes. This tactile reminder allows you to hold a piece of their memory in your hand whenever you need comfort.

In our digital age, creating a website or social media page dedicated to your loved one's memory provides a central place for family and friends to share photos, stories, and memories. This virtual memorial helps you and your family connect and remember them, regardless of physical distance.

Sharing Their Story

Sharing your loved one's story keeps their memory alive while providing support and inspiration to others facing similar challenges.

Writing a memoir or biography documenting your loved one's life story, including their experiences with dementia, preserves their legacy for future generations. This project allows you to process your own emotions while creating a lasting tribute to their life and impact.

Speaking at support groups about your experiences and the lessons you've learned offers valuable insights and comfort to others on similar experiences. Your story can provide hope, practical advice, and a feeling of connection for those now caring for loved ones with dementia.

Starting a blog or video channel to share your progress through grief and remembrance creates a therapeutic outlet for you and a source of connection for others. By openly discussing your experiences, you help break the silence around grief and dementia, fostering a supportive community.

Participating in dementia awareness events, such as walks or runs, honors your loved one's memory while raising awareness and funds for new research. These events often provide a shared sense of community and shared purpose, connecting you with others who understand your experience.

Creating a photo essay or documentary using photographs or video to tell your loved one's story visually captures their essence in a powerful way. This project allows you to revisit cherished memories while creating a lasting tribute to share with others.

Finding Gratitude for Shared Love

Grief at this stage can feel overwhelming, but cultivating gratitude for the love you shared promotes healing and transformation.

Here are five ways to nurture gratitude:

1. **Gratitude Journal**: Regularly write down things you're grateful for about your loved one and your relationship. Include specific memories that bring you joy, lessons they taught you, and ways they positively impacted your life. This practice helps shift your focus to the gifts of your relationship, even amidst loss.

2. **Letter of Thanks**: Write a heartfelt letter to your loved one, expressing your gratitude for their presence in your life. Reflect

on the qualities you admired, the support they provided, and the moments you'll always cherish. This cathartic exercise allows you to articulate your feelings and create a tangible expression of your love and appreciation.

3. **Pay It Forward**: Honor your loved one's memory by extending kindness to others in ways that reflect the love they showed you. Volunteer at a local nursing home, mentor a young person, or help a neighbor in need. By embodying the qualities you admired in your loved one, you keep their spirit alive and spread positivity in the world.

4. **Gratitude Ritual**: Incorporate a daily or weekly gratitude practice into your routine. Light a candle and spend a few moments in quiet reflection on the gifts your loved one brought to your life. This simple ritual provides structure and comfort during times of grief, training your mind to recognize the positive aspects of your relationship.

5. **Celebrate Their Legacy**: Take time to acknowledge and celebrate the positive impact your loved one had on the world around them. Share stories of their kindness with others, continue charitable work they were passionate about, or recognize how their values and teachings continue to shape your life. Focusing on their lasting impact helps you find meaning and purpose in carrying forward their legacy.

Write

Writing about your loved one can be a powerful tool for processing emotions and preserving memories. Consider keeping a journal to record stories, thoughts, and feelings about your loved one. This can become a treasured keepsake for future generations, offering insights into your relationship and your loved one's personality.

You might also consider writing a memoir or a collection of short stories inspired by your loved one's life, to explore their experiences in depth and share their story with a wider audience. Even if you don't intend to publish, the act of writing can be therapeutic and help you maintain a feeling of connection.

Music

Music has a unique ability to evoke memories and emotions. Compile a playlist of your loved ones' favorite songs. Listening to this music can help you feel connected to them and transport you back to shared moments. If you're musically inclined, consider writing a song in their honor. This can be a beautiful and personal tribute, allowing you to express your feelings through melody and lyrics. Even if you're not a professional musician, the act of creating music inspired by your loved one can be deeply meaningful.

Annual Donation

Making an annual donation to a relevant charity on behalf of your loved one continues their impact on causes they cared about. You might choose a different charity each year that aligns with their interests or values.

This practice honors your loved one's memory and allows you to make a positive difference in their name. It can provide a feeling of purpose and continuity in your remembrance activities.

Memory Box

A memory box filled with items that represent different aspects of your loved one's life can be a powerful tool for reminiscence. This can include photos, small objects, letters, or anything else that holds significance.

A memory box can be especially helpful for engaging with someone in the later stages of dementia. The tactile nature of the objects can sometimes spark memories or provide comfort even when verbal communication becomes difficult.

Other Creative Ways to Keep Their Memory Alive

Beyond traditional methods of remembrance, many creative approaches exist to honor your loved one's memory and keep their spirit alive in your daily life.

Memory Recipes: Create a cookbook featuring your loved ones' favorite recipes or dishes they were known for. Include stories or memories associated with each recipe, turning it into a culinary progress through their life. Cooking these dishes allows you to connect with their memory through taste and smell, powerful triggers for emotional memories.

Charitable Giving: Set up a recurring donation to a cause your loved one cared about. This ongoing tribute confirms their values continue to make a positive impact in the world.

Consider involving family members to make it a collective effort, strengthening your bonds through shared remembrance.

Memory Time Capsule: Create a time capsule filled with items representing your loved ones' life and interests. Include letters from family members, photographs, and small mementos.

Set a date in the future to open it together, providing an opportunity for future generations to connect with their legacy.

Memory Bench or Tree: Dedicate a public bench or plant a tree in a meaningful location, finish with a plaque honoring your loved one. This creates a lasting tribute in a place others can enjoy, spreading the positive impact of their memory beyond your immediate circle.

Avoiding Common Pitfalls, Problems and Issues,

I cannot stress this enough: In your efforts to honor your loved one, **don't forget to take care of yourself.**

Balance remembrance activities with self-care and other aspects of your life.

Self-care ensures that you have the emotional resources to continue honoring your loved one's memory in meaningful ways.

While involving others in remembrance activities can be helpful, be mindful that everyone grieves differently.

Don't force participation if others aren't ready or willing.

Respect personal grieving processes and allow space for different forms of remembrance.

Be cautious about letting remembrance activities prevent you from moving forward in your own life. Seek professional help if you find yourself unable to cope with your loss.

That therapist or grief counselor we discussed earlier can also provide valuable support and guidance for others in the grieving process.

Be realistic about what you can manage in terms of remembrance activities. It's better to have a few meaningful practices than to over-commit and feel overwhelmed. Choose activities that truly resonate with you and that you can sustain over time.

Keeping the memory of your loved one alive is a deeply personal concept. Whether through creating tangible reminders, establishing meaningful rituals, sharing their story, or practicing gratitude, these acts of remembrance provide comfort, healing, and a continued sense of connection.

Choose the methods that resonate most with you and that best celebrate the unique person your loved one was and continues to be in your heart.

As you move forward, know that by keeping their memory alive, you're honoring your loved one and preserving an important part of yourself and your shared history.

The goal is to carry the essence of your loved one with you as you continue with your own life. Let their memory inspire you, comfort you, and guide you as you move forward in your life. In doing so, you improve your grief into a lasting tribute to the love you shared.

To Honor Their Memory, Embrace Life Fully

Keeping your loved one's memory alive after their struggle with dementia has ended is a deeply personal and ongoing process. By engaging in meaningful rituals, sharing their story, and finding gratitude for the love you shared, you honor their legacy and find comfort in your memories.

There's no "right" way to remember someone. The most important thing is that your chosen methods feel authentic and meaningful to you.

Be gentle with yourself and allow space that validates both grief and fond remembrance.

Your loved one's impact on your life continues, and by keeping their memory alive, you confirm that their spirit lives on through the love and lessons they shared with you.

Embrace life fully, carrying their memory with you as you create new experiences and connections. This approach honors their legacy by living with the same zest and love they showed during their life.

Your path of remembrance is unique, evolving as you move forward while keeping their spirit close to your heart.

CHAPTER SUMMARY

20 Keys to Keeping Your Loved One's Memory Alive

1. **Create a memory book with photos and mementos.** Gather images, keepsakes, and stories to compile a tangible record of your loved one's life. This serves as a source of comfort and a tool for reminiscence.

2. **Establish annual celebrations to honor their life.** Choose a significant date to host gatherings or events that celebrate your loved one. This provides a regular opportunity for shared remembrance.

3. **Incorporate daily or weekly rituals into your routine.** Light a candle, play their favorite music, or wear a meaningful item regularly. These small acts keep your loved one's presence alive in your daily life.

4. **Use art to express your memories and emotions.** Create collages, quilts, or sculptures using your loved one's belongings or photos. This process can be deeply therapeutic and result in a meaningful tribute.

5. **Write about your loved one's life and your experiences.** Keep a journal, write a memoir, or compose poetry inspired by your loved one. Writing helps process emotions and preserves memories for future generations.

6. **Compile a playlist of their favorite songs.** Music evokes powerful memories and emotions. Listening to your loved one's favorite songs can help you feel connected to them.

7. **Volunteer for causes your loved one cared about.** Dedicate time to organizations or issues that were important to your loved one. This honors their values and continues their legacy of care.

8. **Establish a scholarship or research grant in their name.** Create a lasting impact by funding education or research related to your loved one's interests or experiences. This extends their influence into the future.

9. **Plant a memory garden with their favorite flowers.** Create a living memorial that changes with the seasons. This provides a peaceful space for reflection and connection to nature.

10. **Compile and share their favorite recipes.** Prepare and share meals that your loved one enjoyed. Food often holds strong emotional connections and can be a way to pass on traditions.

11. **Make annual donations to relevant charities.** Choose organizations that align with your loved one's values or interests. This continues their impact on causes they cared about.

12. **Create a memory box of significant items.** Fill a box with objects that represent different aspects of your loved one's life. This can be especially helpful for engaging with someone in later stages of dementia.

13. **Set up a digital memorial or tribute page.** Use websites or social media to share stories and photos of your loved one. This creates an accessible archive for family and friends to contribute to and visit.

14. **Speak at events to share your loved one's story.** Offer to talk at dementia awareness events or support groups. Sharing your experiences can help others and keep your loved one's memory alive.

15. **Start a gratitude journal focused on your loved one.** Write down one thing each day that you're grateful for about your loved one or your relationship. This helps maintain a positive focus amidst grief.

16. **Create a scholarship or fund in their honor.** Establish an educational opportunity or community fund that reflects your loved ones' values. This creates a lasting legacy in their name.

17. **Use their belongings to create functional keepsakes.** Transform clothing into quilts or jewelry into new pieces. These items serve as daily reminders of your loved one.

18. **Record and preserve family stories and histories.** Interview family members and compile a record of your loved one's life and impact. This preserves their legacy for future generations.

19. **Participate in charity events related to their interests.** Join walks, runs, or other fundraisers that align with causes your loved one supported. This combines honoring their memory with making a positive impact.

20. **Create new traditions inspired by their life.** Develop new family customs or activities based on your loved one's interests or values.

This keeps their influence alive in evolving ways.

Love and Letting Go

Loving someone with dementia is a profound testament to the resilience of the human spirit.

This path is filled with challenges, heartache, and unexpected moments of joy.

The blueprint that leads towards caring for someone with dementia is complex and multifaceted, often requiring caregivers to deal with a wide range of emotions while adapting to the changing needs of their loved one.

These challenges can include managing behavioral changes, ensuring safety, and maintaining connection despite cognitive decline.

The complex emotions, practical hurdles, and transformative experiences that come with caring for a loved one whose cognitive abilities are gradually slipping away shape both the caregiver and the person receiving care in profound ways.

Caregivers may experience a range of emotions, including grief, frustration, and guilt, while also developing new skills and deepening their capacity for compassion and patience.

I think that throughout this book, you've found that even though your loved one may suffer from dementia ... while experiencing cognitive decline, may still retain their ability to feel emotions and respond to love and care.

Often in ways that surprise and touch their caregivers deeply.

Let's look over everything we've gone over so far, and close things off with the important lessons we should take with us moving forward:

The Paradox of Dementia Care

Caring for someone with dementia involves an emotional tug-of-war.

You're driven by an overwhelming want to protect and cherish your loved one, yet constantly reminded of the inevitable loss looming on the horizon.

This paradox can manifest in various ways, such as feeling joy when your loved one has a moment of clarity, followed by sadness when they struggle to remember basic information.

It's important to acknowledge and accept these conflicting emotions as a normal part of the caregiving experience. This duality can be exhausting, but it's precisely what makes this experience so deeply human.

The ability to hold space for both love and loss, joy and sorrow, is a uniquely human capacity that can lead to profound personal growth and a deeper understanding of the human condition.

"Grief is the price we pay for love." - *Queen Elizabeth II*

This sentiment pretty much sums up the bittersweet reality of dementia care.

The depth of your pain reflects the strength of your connection.

There's an intrinsic link between love and loss—the pain we feel when losing someone is directly proportional to the love we shared with them.

In the context of dementia care, this can help caregivers reframe their grief as a reflection of their deep love and commitment. By accepting this truth, you can begin to view your grief not as a burden, but as a testament to the meaningful bonds you've forged.

This shift in perspective can be healing, allowing caregivers to honor their pain while also celebrating the love that underlies it.

Be aware that this acceptance is often a process as opposed to a single moment of realization, and it's okay to struggle with this concept at times.

Such an existence might spare you the anguish of grief, but it would also rob you of the joy, growth, and meaning that come from loving deeply.

This hypothetical scenario underscores the value of emotional connections, even when they come with the potential for pain. It suggests that a life lived fully, with all its ups and downs, is ultimately more rewarding than one lived in emotional isolation.

By embracing both the good and bad of this process, you honor the fullness of your human experience. This means acknowledging and accepting all aspects of the caregiving experience, including the difficult moments, those of joy, and everything in between.

It's about recognizing that each experience, whether positive or negative, contributes to your growth and understanding as a caregiver and as a human being.

Vulnerability

One of the most valuable lessons in dementia care is the strength found in vulnerability. When you allow yourself to be vulnerable—to cry, to ask for help, to admit you're not okay—you create space for authentic connections.

Vulnerability in this context doesn't mean weakness—rather, this involves having the courage to be open about your struggles and needs. This openness can lead to deeper, more meaningful relationships and a stronger support network.

By acknowledging your own challenges and emotions, you create an environment where others feel comfortable sharing their own experiences, fostering mutual understanding and empathy.

You give others permission to do the same, fostering a community of support and understanding. By being vulnerable, you create an environment where others feel safe to express their own struggles and emotions.

This reciprocal sharing can help break down barriers of isolation that often accompany caregiving, allowing for a more open and supportive community. It can also foster a proper emotional support system where caregivers can share experiences, offer advice, and provide emotional support to one another. Such a system can be invaluable, especially when facing the challenges of dementia care, offering practical solutions, emotional comfort, and a shared experience that can significantly reduce feelings of isolation and overwhelm.

Research has shown that caregivers who receive social support experience fewer depressive symptoms and better psychological well-being. A comprehensive meta-analysis of 78 studies found that higher levels of perceived social support were associated with lower levels of depression in caregivers.

This research underscores the importance of building and maintaining social connections throughout the caregiving, highlighting how important it is for caregivers to actively seek and nurture supportive relationships.

Social support can come in many forms, including emotional support, practical assistance, and informational resources. Emotional support might involve having someone to talk to about your feelings and experiences.

Practical assistance could include help with caregiving tasks or daily chores.

Informational resources might involve sharing knowledge about dementia care strategies or available services.

Seeking help is a courageous act of self-care and an acknowledgment of our shared humanity. Whether it's joining a support group, talking to a therapist, or confiding in a friend, reaching out can provide invaluable comfort and perspective.

These actions provide immediate relief and contribute to long-term resilience and well-being.

Always remember the importance of seeking help, that it's not a sign of failure or weakness, but rather a proactive step towards better care for both yourself and your loved one with dementia.

By taking care of your own emotional and physical needs, you're better equipped to provide quality care and maintain a positive relationship with your loved one.

Finding Meaning

As you navigate the challenges of loving someone with dementia, it's natural to question the purpose of your suffering. While there are no easy answers, many find that the process of seeking itself becomes a source of profound personal growth and meaning.

Finding meaning can be a powerful coping mechanism, helping to reframe the difficulties of caregiving into opportunities for personal development and deeper understanding. By shifting perspective, caregivers can transform their experience from one of loss and frustration to one of growth and discovery.

This reframing doesn't negate the challenges, but it can provide a new feeling of purpose that makes them more bearable.

Through caregiving, you often explore reserves of strength, compassion, and resilience you never knew you possessed.

Caregiving for someone with dementia often pushes individuals to their limits, revealing inner resources they may not have been aware of. This self-discovery can be both challenging and empowering, leading to personal growth that extends far beyond the caregiving role.

You learn to find joy in small moments, to appreciate the present, and to value the essence of your relationships beyond memory or cognition. This shift in perspective can lead to a deeper appreciation of life and relationships, even in the face of loss and change.

As dementia progresses, caregivers often find themselves focusing on the quality of moments as opposed to their quantity, learning to cherish brief instances of connection or lucidity. This mindfulness practice can profoundly impact your overall outlook on life.

It can also inspire you to become an advocate, raise awareness about dementia, or support others facing similar challenges. By transforming your pain into purpose, you honor your loved one and contribute to a more compassionate and understanding world.

Many caregivers find that sharing their experiences and knowledge helps them process their own experiences while providing valuable support to others. This can include participating in support groups, volunteering with dementia organizations, or even writing about their experiences.

This transformation can provide a feeling of meaning and continuity, allowing the challenges you've faced to benefit others and create positive change.

By finding ways to use their experiences to help others, caregivers can create a lasting legacy that extends beyond their immediate caregiving role, providing purpose that can be particularly comforting as the caregiving phase concludes.

The Role of Technology in Dementia Care

Technology is playing an increasingly important role in dementia care, offering tools to enhance safety, improve quality of life, and support caregivers. While it's not a substitute for human care and connection, technology can be a valuable ally.

The rapid advancement of technology is continually expanding the options available to support patients and their caregivers.

Safety-focused technologies are among the most widely used.

These include GPS tracking devices to prevent wandering, smart home systems for monitoring movement and detecting falls, medication reminders and dispensers, and stove shut-off devices to prevent accidents.

These tools can provide peace of mind for caregivers and allow those with dementia to maintain independence for longer.

For example, GPS tracking devices can allow a person with dementia to continue going for walks independently while providing reassurance to caregivers that they can be located if they become disoriented.

Cognitive stimulation and engagement technologies are also gaining popularity. These include interactive games and puzzles designed for sufferers of dementia, virtual reality experiences that provide sensory stimulation and reminiscence therapy, and robotic companions that offer social interaction and emotional support.

While these technologies can't replace human interaction, they can provide extra stimulation and engagement, particularly during times when caregivers need a break.

For instance, virtual reality programs can allow those with dementia to revisit familiar places or experience new environments safely, potentially triggering positive memories and emotions.

Communication technologies are improving connections between those with dementia, their caregivers, and healthcare providers. Video calling platforms, for instance, can help maintain social connections with distant family members.

Telemedicine services are making it easier to access healthcare without the stress of in-person visits.

These technologies can be particularly beneficial for those with dementia who live in rural areas or have mobility issues that make travel difficult.

Caregiver support technologies are also emerging. These include apps for care coordination, online support groups, and digital platforms for accessing information and resources. These tools can help caregivers feel more connected and supported in their roles.

For example, care coordination apps can help many family members stay informed about their loved one's care needs and share responsibilities more effectively.

While technology offers many benefits, it's important to approach its use thoughtfully. Not all technologies will be suitable or beneficial for every person with dementia.

It's important to consider your loved one's preferences, abilities, and comfort level with technology. Some with dementia may find certain technologies confusing or distressing, while others may adapt to them easily.

Privacy and ethical concerns should also be carefully weighed, particularly with monitoring technologies. The goal should always be to enhance the person's quality of life and support their dignity, not to restrict or control them.

It's important to balance safety concerns with the person's right to privacy and autonomy.

As technology continues to advance, we can expect to see even more innovative solutions for dementia care. However, it's important to remember that technology should complement, not replace, human care and connection.

The most effective dementia care will always involve a balance of technological support and compassionate human interaction.

The Continuum of Love

Love doesn't end with a diagnosis or even with death. The love you share with your family member continues to advance, taking on new forms and expressions as the disease progresses.

This paradigm of love as an evolving, enduring force can be a powerful source of comfort and strength for us caregivers ... it certainly has been for me.

Understanding love as a continuum can provide comfort and purpose throughout the caregiving process and beyond. Recognizing that love can adapt and change as opposed to diminish can help caregivers feel connected in spite of everything, even as their loved one's mental state declines.

In the early stages, your love might manifest as active caregiving and creating new memories. As the disease progresses, it might shift to finding joy in simple presence, touch, or shared silence. These evolving expressions of love can help the feelings of isolation and loneliness that stem from anticipatory grief.

Caregivers often find that nonverbal forms of communication, such as holding hands or listening to music together, become increasingly important as verbal communication becomes more challenging.

Even after your loved one has passed, your love continues through memory, legacy, and the ways you've been transformed by the experience. This ongoing connection can provide comfort and continuity, allowing the relationship to continue to influence and enrich your life.

Many caregivers find that the lessons learned, and personal growth experienced during caregiving continue to shape their lives long after their loved one has passed. These practices can help integrate the loss into your ongoing life narrative.

As you continue this path, may you find strength in your vulnerability, purpose in your pain, and hope in the face of loss. Your love and dedication are making a difference, even when progress is hard to see.

The impact of your care extends far beyond what may be immediately visible, influencing your loved one's quality of life and your own personal growth and the broader understanding of dementia care in society.

A Request

Thank you for taking the time to walk this journey with me.

If this book offered you comfort, insight, or simply reminded you that you're not alone, I'd be so grateful if you shared your thoughts in a review on Amazon. Your words can help others who are searching for support find this book when they need it most.

Thank you, truly, for being part of this story.

Bibliography

1.   Fekete, M., Fekete, M., Lehoczki, A., Lehoczki, A., Tarantini, S., Tarantini, S., Fazekas-Pongor, V., Csípő, T., & Csizmadia, Z. (2023). Improving Cognitive Function with Nutritional Supplements in Aging: A Comprehensive Narrative Review of Clinical Studies Investigating the Effects of Vitamins, Minerals, Antioxidants, and Other Dietary Supplements. Nutrients, 15(24), 5116.

2.   Common Alzheimer's and Dementia Behaviors: Wandering - Caregiver Support & Resources. https://caregiversupportandresources.com/alzheimers-and-dementia-behaviors-wandering/

3.   Experiencing Grief: Navigating the Path to Healing – Evermore Keepsakes. https://evermorekeepsakes.com/blogs/evermore-keepsakes-blog/experiencing-grief-navigating-the-path-to-healing

4.   Expressing Your Grief: Healing Through Writing | TAPS. https://www.taps.org/articles/28-1/healing-through-writing

5.   Budget Pensioners: How to Save Money and Maximize Retirement Income. https://canpension.ca/articles/budget-measures-for-pensioners-ensuring-adequate-support-for-senior-citizens

6.   Top 4 Factors Influencing the Cost of Dementia Care. https://www.desertspringshealthcare.com/resources/cost-of-dementia-care

7.   Finding Balance: The Vital Role of Respite Care for Family Caregivers | Nacifoul. https://nacifoul.com/finding-balance-the-vital-role-of-respite-care-for-family-caregivers/

8.   Experiencing Grief: Navigating the Path to Healing – Evermore Keepsakes. https://evermorekeepsakes.com/blogs/evermore-keepsakes-blog/experiencing-grief-navigating-the-path-to-healing

9.   Essential Tips For Caring For a Spouse With Alzheimer's Disease. https://millerestateandelderlaw.com/9-essential-tips-for-caring-for-a-spouse-with-alzheimers-disease/

10.   Mind Over Matter: Navigating Mental Health Goals in 2025. https://www.openmindwellness.com/post/mind-over-matter-navigating-mental-health-goals-in-2025

11.   What IS Dementia? - Slate Disharoon Parrish and Associates. https://sdp-planning.com/what-is-dementia/

12.   Ways to Support a Loved One with Mental Health Issues: Compassionate Steps for Healing Together - Aspire Atlas. https://aspireatlas.com/10-ways-to-support-a-loved-one-with-mental-health-issues

Appendices

APPENDIX A:
Essential Resources for Dementia Caregivers

Recommended Books

- "The 36-Hour Day" by Nancy L. Mace and Peter V. Rabins

- "Creating Moments of Joy" by Jolene Brackey

- "Learning to Speak Alzheimer's" by Joanne Koenig Coste

- "The Dementia Caregiver's Little Book of Hope" by Patricia Smith

- "When Reasoning No Longer Works" by Angel Smits

Support Groups & Organizations

- Family Caregiver Alliance (www.caregiver.org)

- National Association of Area Agencies on Aging (www.n4a.org)

- Local memory cafés and support groups

- Alzheimer's Association (www.alz.org)

    o   24/7 Helpline: 1-800-272-3900

    o   Local chapter finder

    o   Online community forums

- Online communities (Facebook groups, Reddit r/dementia)

Conversation Starters

Reminiscence Topics

Childhood Memories

- "Tell me about your favorite childhood game"
- "What was your family home like?"
- "Who was your best friend growing up?"
- "What did you like best about school?"

Life Achievements

- "What was your first job?"
- "Tell me about your wedding day"
- "What are you most proud of?"

Simple Pleasures

- "What's your favorite season?"
- "Do you enjoy listening to music?"
- "What's your favorite food?"
- "Do you like sports or art?"
- "Who is your favorite movie star?"

Activity-Based Conversations

Photo Albums

- "Who is this in the picture?"
- "Where was this taken?"

- "What was happening that day?"

Nature

- "Look at those beautiful flowers - which color do you like best?"

- "Do you hear the birds singing?"

- "How does the sunshine feel?"

Music

- "Would you like to listen to some music?"

- "Did you ever dance to this song?"

- "What kind of music makes you happy?"

Remember: Keep conversations simple, positive, and focused on one topic at a time. Use short sentences and give plenty of time for responses.

About the Author

Nadia Wells is the author of Grieving the Living: Coping with Grief and Loss While Loving Someone with Dementia, a heartfelt guide born from personal experience and a deep desire to help others navigate the emotional complexities of dementia caregiving.

When Nadia's father was diagnosed with dementia, she found herself walking a path filled with love, heartache, and unspoken grief. Through that journey, she discovered the power of shared stories, compassionate support, and everyday moments of connection.

Determined to turn her experience into something meaningful, Nadia spent countless hours researching, interviewing healthcare professionals and grief counselors, and engaging with others in dementia support groups.

Her writing blends personal insight with practical guidance, offering caregivers a gentle companion through one of life's most difficult seasons. With this book, Nadia hopes to remind readers that while dementia may take many things, it cannot erase love—and no one should face this journey alone.

About the Publisher

At JMCG Press, we are passionate about storytelling and ideas that inspire, inform, and entertain. As an independent publisher, we embrace diverse voices and genres, curating books that spark curiosity and create meaningful connections with readers. From thought-provoking non-fiction to immersive fiction and everything in between, our mission is to bring fresh perspectives to the page and to the world.

Your support means everything to us! If you've enjoyed one of our books, please consider leaving a review. Your feedback not only helps our authors thrive but also empowers small publishers like us to continue championing creativity and unique stories. Thank you for being part of our journey!

www.ingramcontent.com/pod-product-compliance
Lightning Source LLC
Chambersburg PA
CBHW070805280326
41934CB00012B/3066